D1562901

SHORT WHITE COAT

Early versions of several chapters have been previously published, and with the kind permission of the following journals, are reproduced herein.

Academic Medicine, "Anaphylactic Shock"
Archives of Pediatrics & Adolescent Medicine, "Setting Sights"
Journal of the American Geriatrics Society, "Her Voice Alone"
Journal of General Internal Medicine, "Bag of Humility"
The New Physician, "Indiscriminate Hands"
The New Physician, "Lift"
The New Physician, "The King and I"

Short
White
Coat

*Lessons from Patients on
Becoming a Doctor*

JAMES A. FEINSTEIN, MD

iUniverse, Inc.
New York Bloomington

Short White Coat
Lessons from Patients on Becoming a Doctor

iUniverse books may be ordered through booksellers or by contacting:

iUniverse
1663 Liberty Drive
Bloomington, IN 47403
www.iuniverse.com
1-800-Authors (1-800-288-4677)

Because of the dynamic nature of the Internet, any Web addresses or links contained in this book may have changed since publication and may no longer be valid.

ISBN: 978-1-4401-7513-8 (sc)
ISBN: 978-1-4401-7515-2 (dj)
ISBN: 978-1-4401-7514-5 (ebk)

Printed in the United States of America

iUniverse rev. date: 10/29/2009

For my parents, my grandmothers, and Amy

Peace. It does not mean to be in a place where there is no noise, trouble, or hard work. It means to be in the midst of those things and still be calm in your heart…

—*Author unknown*

CONTENTS

SURGERY

EMERGENCY MEDICINE

PREFACE

M Y THIRD YEAR of medical school—the clinical year of medical school—was like most things in life that have caused me to mature internally. Before I could enjoy the validation of knowing I probably could make a career in this profession called "doctoring," I first had to survive the rites of initiation that every medical student faces. After finishing the second year of medical school, I was required to shed my bookworm cocoon and replace it with a pristine, too-short white coat. The short white coat has come to epitomize the role of the medical student: the coat is barely long and functional enough to carry all the educational books and tools of a medical student, but plenty short and awkward enough to remind any onlooker of the partially hatched novice contained within. The transition from learning in a classroom to working in a hospital occurs overnight, and it is not an easy or painless switch. One day I sat in a lecture hall memorizing the intricacies of mitochondrial metabolism, and the next day I showed up for morning rounds terrified by the prospect of caring for living and breathing people.

This rapid transformation that takes place during the third year of medical school requires medical students to confront the many "firsts" of becoming a doctor in a head-on, no-holds-barred, full-contact kind of way. Over the course of the year, I learned how doctors cared for patients. I applied this newfound knowledge, and I too learned patient care, though usually not until I had tried many different approaches to find what worked.

Throughout the process, I experienced my fair share of missteps, second guesses, uncertainties, and embarrassments. More often than not, these things caused me to ponder that nagging question that plagues every medical student at least a few times during the four years of medical school: "Do I have what it takes to become a doctor?"

Oddly enough, it was exactly those uncertainties, more than anything I could have learned from a textbook, that truly taught me how to help people. At first, what I had to offer my patients were the simple and non-medical things that it seemed like anyone could have provided. I learned how to fetch a newspaper, adjust a bedside tray table, regurgitate a list of lab values for the medical team, or—in the spirit of my Montessori school days— neatly clip the ends of the glorified strings commonly referred to as "sutures." Then, as I began to gain a footing and find my place in the hospital, I increasingly functioned as a contributing member of a medical team. I learned how to take a patient's history, discuss medication interactions with the pharmacist, make an incision into human flesh, or—what I still consider the greatest privilege given to a medical student—deliver a baby.

The amazing thing about this trial-by-fire system of medical education is that by the time I had a moment to pick up my head and survey everything I had experienced during my third year of medical school, by the time I was in a position to answer that question of questions, it was too late. I no longer wondered why the medical school admissions committee had graciously let any of my fellow classmates or me into medical school. Without exception, we had all grown into our ill-fitting, too-short white coats, and we would soon outgrow them altogether.

During my tenure in caring for people and their health, I've realized that the process of becoming a doctor—and ultimately being a doctor—involves a great deal of patience, humility, and, more than anything else, the ability and the desire to say: "I don't know, but I am going to try to figure it out." The answer might be as deceivingly simple as fiddling to adjust the height of a patient's tray table, or it might be as dauntingly complex as sorting through a patient's myriad symptoms to make a diagnosis. In the end, it's that innate drive to figure out how best to help people that makes all those other things—the things that made me question my decision to become a doctor—fade into the background. It doesn't mean that the difficulties associated with the "firsts" aren't valid. After all, they did fill the following pages of this book. Rather, I believe that those experiences—the good and the bad— are necessary steps in learning the art of doctoring.

James A. Feinstein, MD

INTERNAL MEDICINE

CHAPTER ONE

LINGO

"CALM DOWN, HONEY. I'm gonna help you, okay? Don't panic. Just tell me what's wrong."

My lip wouldn't stop quivering. My whole body tingled with fear. I wanted to turn around, run beyond the double swinging doors out into the open, and gulp down the cold winter air. I didn't, though. For some reason, I trusted the operator's voice on the other end of the receiver.

"Listen. This is what I want you to do."

At least a half-dozen times before I arrived at this point of terror, I had attempted to page my resident according to the instructions I had scribbled down on a crumpled piece of paper. Nevertheless, each time I entered the number, the phone spit back an angry tone, signaling that I'd done something to provoke the paging system. Realizing that I was going to be late on my first day working as a medical student in the hospital, I surrendered and called the switchboard operator to help bail me out of my mess. I thought, "I've been in the hospital less than five minutes, and I have already become the patient."

The previous night, I had fallen asleep expecting to wake up and start learning the business of improving people's health, but I couldn't affect people's lives without knowing how to find them. In those moments before the voice rescued me, I had fast-forwarded to the end of the day, imagining myself still sitting in the same place, while the rest of the new medical team left the hospital after a long day of treating patients. I could almost see the quizzical looks on their faces, wondering why I—their new medical student—hadn't shown up. "He didn't know how to use his pager," the clerkship director would explain to the dean of the medical school. "He needs remediation."

The operator's soothing voice brought me back to the task.

"Punch the pound sign, eight, and then one into the keypad. This will connect you to the hospital's paging system. Can you hear the paging menu, honey?"

I followed the voice's calm directions. If the first two years of medical school had taught me anything, it was how to follow instructions. I had spent countless hours memorizing and then regurgitating chemical pathways, lists of symptoms, and treatment flowcharts. Now, it seemed like those hours had anything but paid off—I could barely dial a telephone number. Maybe those lists of diseases and symptoms and drugs had bullied away the street-smart savvy on which I used to pride myself. Regardless, I understood that nothing—not even my practical intuition—could have prepared me for my frightening, first moments in the hospital.

"Now I want you to press four to send a page. Okay?"

I keyed the number four into the phone and waited.

"Perfect. You're doing okay. Now enter your resident's pager number. Then your number. And then—this is the most important part—press the pound sign at the end to make sure to send the page. You should hear a beeping noise if it went through correctly. Do you hear it?"

I did. Then I exhaled for the first time since the operator's voice had begun to guide me through my crisis.

"Thank you, thank you, thank you," I said, in exchange for the kind woman's help.

Then, as quickly as I had let my mind spin out of control with fear, I regained my composure and felt a surge of relief rush through my body. My lower lip quit quivering. Certain that the incident had been a fluke, I felt ready to continue with the business of changing lives.

While I waited for my supervising resident to appear, I lingered near the counter of the nurses' station. I tried to look confident, like I belonged there. Somehow, after my mishap with the pager, I couldn't calm the nervous feeling in the pit of my stomach. It didn't help that the new sights and smells and sounds of the hospital made every one of my senses uncomfortable. The rough, starched collar of my short white coat chafed at my neck. I could feel the crunch of the impeccably white fabric as I leaned against the counter. My deep pockets overflowed with medical instruments, cards with different lists of symptoms and therapies, and even a mini-textbook. Because of the weight of the pockets, I felt like I had a yoke around my neck. Every so often, someone rushed by and the resulting movement of air replaced the sharp, sanitized smell of the hospital ward with the unmistakable stench of human urine and feces. Mostly, though, I focused on the buzzing noise of a hospital whirring to life while I waited for my resident to welcome me.

Instead, a frustrated, almost angry voice punctuated the drone of the bustling doctors and nurses. A tall woman in a long white coat walked toward me, and I assumed she was my new supervising resident.

"Why didn't you answer the phone when I returned your page?"

It took me a few moments before I realized that the words had been directed toward me. Even then, I didn't quite grasp the meaning. I *had* paged my resident. I hadn't done anything wrong. The resident rephrased her question, turning it into my second lesson of the day about the nuances of paging.

"You're supposed to pick up the phone when someone returns a page! Didn't you hear the nurses on the loudspeaker system asking whoever paged me to pick up the phone? How the hell am I supposed to find you otherwise?"

I realized that I'd completely ignored that when you page someone, only the phone number shows up on the page—not a message, a location, or a name.

"You're lucky that I recognized you," she scoffed.

Although I was thankful she'd found me before rounds began, I also understood the silent message in her comment: "I spotted you from a mile away. How could I miss you in your short white coat with your idiotic, bulging pockets?" Before I could consider this further, the resident took off in full stride down the hallway. I hurried to catch up with her, and as we rounded a corner, several other flashes of white now moved in sync with the two of us. My first rounding experience had officially begun.

—⊷—

The first visit of the morning brought us to the room of Andre Benson, an octogenarian who scowled at the medical team through his doorway. The resident cryptically began to recount the events of Mr. Benson's previous night in the hospital.

"Eighty-one-year-old male with history of alcoholism presents with DVT and PE. No shortness of breath or dyspnea. Significant lower extremity swelling. No pain overnight. Patient taking adequate PO's. PT and INR are subtherapeutic. Plan is to keep in-house until anticoagulated."

She finished presenting her succinct update, and I could only remember that "PT" translated to prothrombin time, a measure of the blood's intrinsic ability to clot. Since PT was the single acronym I recognized during her entire presentation, I tried to peek through the doorway and visually assess for myself why Mr. Benson had ended up in the hospital. I couldn't see anything but his now sullen face poking out from underneath the layers of hospital blankets, and by the time I had turned my attention back to the team, they had moved on to another room.

Once again, I jogged down the hallway, my pockets swinging with each stride, and I tried to decode and process the remainder of the resident's assessment of Mr. Benson's health. I wondered how I would ever survive the next hour of rounds, if for no other reason than I was not physically fit enough to keep up with the rest of the Olympic-fast team.

———

When I started medical school two years earlier, no one told me it would be the most difficult experience of my life. Although my senior classmates had acknowledged that the first two years of basic science courses would shake the most confident student, this was always trumped by the notion that the final two years—the in-hospital, clinical years—would make everything worthwhile. "When you stand in front of a patient, all those hours of memorizing and cramming will pay off," they had said, unanimously.

Indeed, they had correctly predicted the course of my first two years of medical school. On several occasions, I found myself basing my self-worth on a few lousy numbers, and I routinely wondered why in the world I had considered myself fit for the medical profession. Only near the end of my second year did I acclimate to the challenging environment, once I learned to place emphasis on the process of learning, rather than on my grades. Unfortunately, just when I started to become comfortable with one topic or experience, the medical education system always managed to drag the rug out from underneath my feet, throw me into a new situation, and leave me feeling overwhelmed and unsettled. I'd just mastered how to dissect a cadaver when we moved on to a completely separate task of learning how to examine a living patient. Even though I'd come to expect these kinds of transitions, I never thought my introduction to working in the hospital would be so jarring.

In the days leading up to that first morning in the hospital, my friends, and family had affirmed that I had arrived at the doorstep of my calling: "You're meant to be around people. You're such a good listener." I was embarrassed for believing their ego-stoking words. I couldn't dial a pager number. I couldn't follow what seemed to be a routine presentation about a patient. I didn't believe I would ever appear—or feel—confident enough to take care of patients. With my pockets swinging as I ran after the team, I somehow felt I deserved my position at the end of the line.

———

Outside the next patient's room, the resident reported to us that the Emergency Room (ER) had just sent the patient, Estelle Grady, to our ward for evaluation of a suspected MI. This time I recognized the abbreviation instantly: myocardial infarction—heart attack. Having just finished the basic science course in cardiology, I was determined to keep up with the discussion.

The resident proceeded to tell us about the patient's past medical history, then the events leading up to Ms. Grady's trip to the ER, completing her presentation with Ms. Grady's laboratory results.

"Her first and second CK's were normal. Her first troponin was zero point three."

These words were more familiar. Even though I didn't know how to interpret the values, at least I recognized the terminology. As we moved on, I walked alongside the rest of the team, and I nodded my head at their comments about Ms. Grady's condition.

After rounds ended, the attending physician—the boss of the team—pulled me aside. I felt certain I was about to receive another lecture on paging etiquette or a directive to go to the gym to get in shape so I could keep up with the medical team on rounds.

"I noticed that you seemed to take an interest in Ms. Grady's case. I think that the workup of a myocardial infarction is good bread-and-butter medicine. Do you want to follow her as your own patient?"

Elated, I could only nod.

"Good. Why don't you follow Mr. Benson, too," the attending physician said. "Oh, and when you go back to see Ms. Grady, tell her that her repeat labs were negative. You can also let her know that as long as the next set comes back negative, we'll plan to send her home tomorrow morning. She'll be able to follow up with her own doctor to monitor her condition."

A surge of purpose rushed through my body as I took off toward Ms. Grady's room.

As I sat by Ms. Grady's bedside, I was determined to figure out the cause of her chest pain. Maybe if I did, I would impress the team enough to make up for my athletic shortcomings earlier that morning. I questioned her about the various things that might have precipitated her chest pain.

"Were you doing anything different when the pain occurred?"

I felt confident as I ran through the list of symptoms that I had memorized during the first two years of medical school.

"How about a history of chest pain or heart trouble?" I continued. "Asthma or breathing problems? Heartburn or reflux?"

Once I completed the interview, I tried my best to perform a cardiac exam on Ms. Grady. I listened to her heart and examined her pulses. Then, as instructed by the attending physician, I began to speak with her about the results of her cardiac laboratory tests. The confidence in my voice surprised me.

"Your last troponin level was zero point three. If your next troponin level is the same, then you might be able to go home tomorrow," I said. I used my most doctor-like voice, and I recited almost word for word what the attending physician had told me.

Instead of a look of relief, I recognized the unmistakable quivering lip of a terrified patient. I had anticipated that the promising test results would put Ms. Grady at ease. It caught me by surprise that she appeared more worried than before. As tears welled up in the corners of her eyes, I panicked. What had I said to make her react in this way?

I uttered the same universal, no-nonsense question the phone operator had asked me just a few hours earlier.

"What's wrong, Ms. Grady?"

After a moment's hesitation, she began to speak.

"Honey, I don't know what 'tronins' are. But you said I have them—zero point three of them. Does that mean that my heart is bad?"

Immediately I realized my mistake: I'd assumed the stereotypical role of a doctor. I was caught up in scientific terminology instead of communicating the information most important to Ms. Grady. I wondered how I had forgotten the helpless feeling I'd experienced that morning while my resident spewed foreign medical terminology.

"I'm so sorry," I said. "Troponin levels help us to identify when a person has had a heart attack. Your troponin level was zero point three and that's completely normal. Everyone has a bit of troponin floating around in their bloodstream, even with a totally healthy heart."

Ms. Grady looked less panicked.

"So, no, your heart isn't bad," I said.

Picking up her dining menu, I drew the rough outline of a heart, illustrating how a heart attack caused the release of little bits of troponin into the bloodstream. Ms. Grady confirmed each of the steps with a "Mm-hmm," and when I finished with my explanation, I noticed that her bottom lip had quit quivering.

Early the next morning, before rounds began, I visited both of my patients to see how they had fared the night. For no particular reason, I decided to visit Mr. Benson first.

"Hey, Doc," he said cautiously as I entered his room.

Almost reflexively, I blurted, "I'm just a medical student, Mr. Benson."

"Medical student. Doctor. Whatever. You're all the same to me—a bunch of shysters. Just tell me how my blood is this morning. Can I go home?"

I had already checked the results of his coagulation profile that morning. Having read up on the subject the previous night, I knew his numbers suggested that his blood thinning medication had yet to kick in. Nonetheless, knowing my current place at the bottom of the chain of command, I swiftly dodged the question.

"I'm not quite sure yet. Your PT is thirteen and your INR is one, but I'm still learning how to interpret the values. It's better if the rest of the team explains what those results mean."

Although unspoken, I think we both realized that Mr. Benson would probably spend many more days lying in wait until the team could discover what had caused the clot in his leg. Upset by my avoidance of his question, he turned back to the blaring television as I sheepishly walked out of the room. I felt like I had deceived Mr. Benson by hiding behind the same abbreviations and numbers that left me confused and unsatisfied the day before.

Ms. Grady's room was a few paces down the hallway. I leafed through her chart, which lay on a counter outside her door. I began to review her vital signs, but before I had the chance to read her laboratory values, I heard her calling from inside her room.

"Good morning, Doc!"

I walked in and found myself correcting her in the same way I had Mr. Benson.

"I'm just a medical student, Ms. Grady."

"You ain't *just* anything," she said. Her radiant face told me that something good had happened since I'd seen her last.

"Honey, my 'tronins' came back normal!"

I matched her smile with one of my own.

"The nurse told me my last level was point zero three. I'm gonna be A-okay."

Me too, I hoped. I squeezed her hand, adding, "The rest of our medical team will be back soon so we can talk about getting you home."

Then I walked out the door, located a phone, and paged my resident, eager to see the remainder of the day's patients.

CHAPTER TWO

ANAPHYLACTIC SHOCK

L IKE BEING IMMERSED in any foreign culture, a week or two in the hospital was all I needed to notice the local customs and practices. Thus far, I had learned that the main responsibilities of a medical student consisted of picking several patients to follow during their hospital stays, presenting these patients' histories to the medical team each morning, and preparing mini-reviews on the most current research regarding these patients' illnesses.

Lore existed among my fellow medical students that these presentations had to be as polished and flawless as a presidential address—our entire medical worth depended on them. At the end of each presentation, the medical team sized up the medical student by asking questions designed to make sure a medical student understood his low rank. This humiliating process directed toward medical students was commonly referred to as "pimping." Thus, in a survival of the fittest kind of way, medical students would gather and hoard patient information so that each one of us might somehow deliver the perfect, complete presentation and achieve the holy grail: a plain and silent nod of approval from the attending physician.

I noticed that each attending physician seemed to have his own set of preferred questions that he asked about a patient's medical history—regardless of the patient's actual symptoms or diagnoses. Some of them wanted an exhaustive account of a patient's past travel history. Others wanted a detailed analysis of a patient's use of seatbelts and bicycle helmets. Given that a new attending physician assumed control of the ship every two weeks, with new residents every four weeks, the possible combinations of their pet preferences seemed dauntingly endless.

As absurd as some of the requests for information sometimes seemed, I nevertheless began to realize that the more patient information I collected up front, the better prepared I would be to answer any questions thrown at me. I turned interviewing patients into a game of collecting every scrap of information. Then, when an attending physician inevitably asked some esoteric question, I could answer coolly and without hesitation.

"Has the patient ever taken a sulfa drug in his whole, entire life?"

"Yes."

"What is the patient's favorite food?"

"Pizza."

"What is her shoe size?"

"Eight."

Amid a sea of constant change, my exhaustive interviewing technique afforded me some protection against an unexpected question.

After introducing myself to Erich Allen, a new and somewhat frightened patient lying before me, I skipped the small talk of introductions, and for the sake of efficiency, launched directly into a full-blown interrogation. I scrolled down my mental checklist, making sure to collect any tidbit of information that the attending physician might deem necessary to Mr. Allen's care. By the end of my cross-examination, he looked completely exhausted. I took the opportunity to excuse myself, and I exited his room so I could get a head start on preparing my presentation.

Later that night, unable to sleep because of an overactive heating vent in my overnight call room, I began to pace the empty hospital hallways while practicing my presentation in my head. I meticulously pieced together the information Mr. Allen had supplied, and I took care to include every relevant fact. By the time rounds began the following morning, I convinced myself that I had perfected a bibliography of Mr. Allen's life so complete that the attending physician wouldn't have to ask a single question.

We approached Mr. Allen's room, and I confidently wove my way to the front of the crowd of long white coats. I cleared my throat and prepared to deliver my presentation. But before I could get any words out, I realized I had forgotten my patient's name. A wave of fear swept through my body. I stood in shock, my heart pounded, and I wondered how I had managed to get myself into this situation. I had been so focused on anticipating the attending physician's questions, that I had lost sight of the patient. My eyes scanned the blank faces attached to the long white coats. They waited. I frantically looked around the room, and my eyes searched for something that might remind me of my patient's name—and then I found it. On Mr. Allen's pale wrist sat a neon orange hospital bracelet, its inscription just barely legible from where I stood. With a renewed confidence, I began to speak.

"Everyone, this is Mr. Shellfish. He is a sixty-two-year-old male with a past history of hypertension, diabetes, and—"

I heard a rumble beside me. I continued reciting his medication list before I realized that Mr. Shellfish had erupted into a giant, full-bellied fit of laughter. His chest heaved beneath the thin, white hospital gown, and his shrieks of amusement filled the room. I couldn't hear anyone else laughing, which perplexed me. Had I forgotten to inquire about a psychiatric history? The patient hadn't seemed delirious that morning during pre-rounds.

I did the only thing I could, and I pushed onward with the presentation. But I stopped once I began to recite the patient's list of allergies—Mr. Allen had an allergy to shellfish.

I stood mortified before the medical team, stuttered for a few moments, and then finished the remainder of my presentation. At the conclusion, I followed the team out of the room with my tail between my legs. As I had done that first day in the hospital, I tossed my visions of residency into the wastebasket next to Mr. Allen's door. Once again, those feelings of inadequacy surfaced. How would I ever take care of multiple patients when I couldn't remember *one* patient's name?

Luckily, the attending physician chose to ignore my blunder. Instead, he began peppering me with questions about Mr. Allen's travel history and his favorite hobbies. The practiced answers rolled off my tongue, although that day the attending physician's affirmative nods failed to excite me. I stood there like a fraud and thought that anyone could have filled my shoes.

After rounds ended, I felt an urgent need to apologize to Mr. Allen. When I walked back into his room, three unfamiliar faces looked up at me. A woman seated at his bedside stood, beamed, and offered me her hand.

"Hi, I'm Mrs. Shellfish and these are our two children," she said, motioning with her hand. The four of them burst into uncontrolled laughter. I cast my eyes downward, smiled sheepishly, and then succumbed to the humor of my mistake. After a few moments of levity, I turned my attention to Mr. Allen and apologized for having forgotten his name. Once he caught his breath, he looked at me and spoke.

"Shhhh. You don't need to apologize for anything, son. I haven't laughed like that in weeks—although I'm sorry that no one else got your joke. Keep it up. You're doing just fine."

I wish I could say I was a completely changed person following that incident, but I wasn't. In my short tenure as a third year medical student, I realized that my instructors would continue to evaluate me on the answers I supplied to some of their innocuous questions. And, because attending physicians were never going to stop asking questions, I still needed to collect every bit of information from a patient, despite having just learned firsthand the inherent dangers in doing so.

The difference in my actions, I realized, needed to occur in the way that I collected the information. During the next several weeks, I deliberately devoted less and less time to crossing off mental checkboxes, and instead, I talked more freely with each of my patients. Not surprisingly, once I made this transition, I found myself learning and remembering more about my patients' lives than I had during my first few weeks in the hospital. While I still wasn't able to answer every obscure question that an attending physician directed at me, I did find myself becoming more comfortable with the phrase, "I don't know"—if for no other reason than because I knew my patients and their names well enough to go back for a friendly visit and find out the answer.

CHAPTER THREE

WAITING

TIME MOVED DIFFERENTLY in the hospital. While it seemed to spiral forward at a breakneck pace for me, it followed a more normal distribution for almost everyone else. Some people, like Mr. Benson with the clots in his legs, arrived in the hospital only to wait and wait for something to happen. The majority of people, like Ms. Grady, settled in for a few days of routine testing, or to recover from a common illness, and then they disappeared back into their normal existences. And the remainder—these were the people whose entire lives changed at the drop of a hat.

Gina Piazzo arrived on the internal medicine floor after spending a long day in the ER. Exhibiting maturity beyond her years, her young daughter had persuaded Gina to drive into the city after witnessing her cough up a spot of blood. The cough had started out innocently enough the previous weekend. But by Monday morning, it had progressed to a full, body-shaking hack. Gina, who kept up-to-date on the media's constant coverage of the raging influenza epidemic, believed that she had been stricken by the flu. She knew enough to realize that a trip to the ER was probably in her best interest, so she and her daughter drove to the hospital.

What Gina didn't know, however, was that ER physicians usually treated an uncomplicated case of pneumonia with powerful antibiotics, and then sent the patient home the same day. Only when a patient had difficulty maintaining the oxygen levels in her blood, or in Gina's case, had a suspicious finding on her chest radiograph, did it warrant an admission to the hospital. The ER physician had discovered a small, quarter-size opacity on her chest film. He explained to Gina that he wanted her to stay overnight so he could perform a few more tests. He wondered why an otherwise healthy young woman had acquired a severe case of pneumonia. He didn't mention anything more, especially not the forbidden word "cancer."

The attending physician on the medicine ward had little doubt that Gina's small mass was anything other than cancer. After presenting the attending physician with Gina's history, I ran through a list of differential diagnoses for a suspicious lung mass. I focused on the rare infectious causes, certain that the culprit in an otherwise healthy young woman *must* be something obscure. It helped that we had studied the rare exceptions in detail during the basic science years—I gave them substantial weight while trying to determine the different causes of Gina's chest mass. But the attending physician had seen a hundred cases similar to Gina's presentation, and she reminded me of one of the more important rules of medicine: "Common things are common. Cancer is common."

Afterward, I remember walking somberly alongside the attending physician into Gina's room. The rest of the team had stayed behind in the hall to make the ensuing conversation as intimate and as nonthreatening as possible. Gina lay in her bed looking wilted beneath her thin hospital gown, and she writhed with each cough. Her mom clothes—a pair of red sweat pants, slip-on shoes, and a diaper bag that revealed she had another small child at home—were piled in the corner.

The young daughter stood beside her mother's bed. The girl's eyes were tearful and wide with fear. I thought back to several weeks before, when the sounds and sights of the hospital had overwhelmed my own senses, and then I tried to picture my mother lying amid this frightening new stimulation—the resulting image terrified me. I was scared for Gina, but more scared for her daughter.

"Why don't you go out in the hallway?" the attending physician said to the young girl. "You can tell the rest of the nice doctors about your favorite things you do at school."

Then, the physician found a place on Gina's bed and sat beside her. She gently placed her hand on Gina's knee. Gina's upper body continued to heave with more coughing.

"I'm sorry that you're feeling so lousy," the attending physician said. "We'll get you some strong cough syrup so you can have a break from this hacking. In the meantime, I want to sit and talk with you a bit. Is that okay? You can just nod—I know that talking right now is kind of painful."

Gina nodded.

"I believe in being up-front with my patients," the attending physician continued. "And I want to be honest with you—I am concerned about the radiograph of your lungs. I'm not sure if anyone went over it with you, but there is a small marking on the radiograph that shouldn't be there."

Gina nodded again.

"I don't want to make you worry too much at this point, but it is unusual. I want to get a CT scan of your lungs. It will give me a better picture of what might be going on."

Gina nodded yet again, and I could see the corners of her eyes swelling with water. She cast her eyes downward and fidgeted with the corner of the hospital blanket. Even without Gina having said anything, I could almost see the word "cancer" bouncing around her mind. The attending physician had a similar sense, and she decided to address the fear straight on.

"We still need to do more testing, but I know you're probably thinking the worst. I've thought about it, too. One of my concerns is that it might be cancer. But there are also other things that we need to rule out before I can give you a definite answer."

The attending physician paused and gave Gina a moment to think.

"I understand how scary this must be. I'm going to do my best to arrange for these tests to be done immediately, so that you don't have to wonder for too long. I know this is a lot all at once, but do you have any questions?"

Gina moved her head from side to side, clearly overwhelmed, while the attending physician sat and rubbed Gina's leg. I thought about how quickly this woman's entire life had turned upside down. Gina's only concerns just a few hours earlier had been about managing the morning chaos of getting two children to school and daycare, making sure that everyone had breakfast and a packed lunch, and starting her own workday on time as a bank teller. Now I imagined her, still concerned about readying her two kids for the day, only this time wondering *who* would be pouring the cereal and slicing the sandwiches and kissing the cheeks if and when she was no longer there.

The team shuffled down the corridor to finish rounding on the remaining patients. We visited with a few people before we reached Mr. Benson's room. After two weeks of sitting in the hospital, our daily interaction with Mr. Benson had been reduced to a courteous social call. We continued to wait for the results of his genetic clotting tests to come back from a national laboratory. Nothing else could be done medically other than hope that his anticoagulation medication might take effect. So each day we poked our heads into his room, ashamed that we had no new news for Mr. Benson, said a brief hello, and then scuttled onward to the next patient's room where we might actually do something.

By this point, Mr. Benson rarely responded to the team's morning visits. His gaze never deviated from the blaring television hanging over the foot of his bed. Perhaps he felt duped. A few days earlier, he had articulated that he could just as easily be waiting in the comfort of his own home.

"If I had known it would turn out this way, I wouldn't have bothered to come in," he said. "I don't care how much pain I was in. It still wouldn't be worth sitting here and watching you shysters *not* do a damn thing for me!"

On some level, I understood his resentment: we had discovered a serious, possibly life-threatening medical condition that needed treatment, but to him it appeared as if we weren't doing anything other than holding him against his will.

Later that evening, once I made it back to the quiet safety of my apartment, I wondered about the unfairness of it all. Gina lay there in fear because the doctors knew too much. Mr. Benson lay in anger because we knew too little. Neither was happy, and yet, they each did the only thing they could—Mr. Benson waited for his life to begin again, and Gina waited for her tragic ending to unfold.

During my workday, I willingly pushed each of their predicaments from the front of my mind. Although I found myself matching their individual paces while in their presence, once I stepped out of either of their rooms, I was off again at a fast pace to collect more lab values, help admit another patient, or run to a lecture. Intuitively, I knew that if I slowed down too much, I might think too much. And if I thought too much, it just might hurt too much.

Chapter Four

Forced Participation

"**D**on't put those there," a stern voice admonished from behind me, while I fumbled to unload the contents of my hands.

Just moments into one of my call nights, at the request of my resident, I had gathered the necessary tubes, needles, and alcohol wipes used to draw blood. A paramedic had just given us a report about a new patient he had transported by ambulance directly from another hospital. The patient had sickle cell disease and needed to have several things done immediately, including some blood tests. Because the phlebotomist had already left for the evening, we had to draw the patient's blood ourselves. Correction—I needed to draw the patient's blood myself.

Once I had dropped the supplies into a pocket on my short white coat, I turned around to see who had delivered the instructions. In the corner of the room, a uniformed police officer sat on a chair tipped back against the wall. He flipped casually through pages of a *People* magazine. I noticed that he had a large gun strapped to his plump waist.

"You can't put needles or sharp things down near the prisoner," he said, not once looking up from his magazine.

I did a double take and looked back toward the patient. At first glance, he appeared no different from anyone else lying in a hospital bed. Then, as I traced the length of his arm with my eyes, I noticed that a gleaming steel handcuff bound his wrist to the hospital bed. His other arm also bore a shackle, and so did one of his legs. He was completely immobilized. Judging by the sight of his pale, sickly face, I couldn't imagine that he would have run off anyway—he looked like he felt horrible.

Despite the presence of the police officer and the handcuffs, I felt uneasy. Wondering what the patient had done to end up in prison, I imagined him as a drug dealer, a burglar, or worse yet, a murderer. I worked myself into a panic thinking about trying to draw blood—something I was already terrible at—from a hardened criminal. I'd seen the movie *Silence of the Lambs*. If I didn't perform perfectly, I imagined that he'd find some way to hunt my family down: "This is payback for the sloppy job your son did while drawing my blood!"

I felt doomed. My short but illustrious blood-drawing career consisted of two awful, scarring experiences. The first time I had drawn blood, I had practiced on one of my unlucky classmates. Although I miraculously punctured the correct vein, I fumbled while trying to connect the collection tube to the needle, which inadvertently moved the needle and caused a giant bruise to form under his skin. By the time I realized what I had done, my fellow medical student had a gigantic, purple contusion spreading across his forearm. It looked incredibly painful and took a full two weeks to heal. My classmates never let me hear the end of it.

After that initial experience, I avoided all subsequent opportunities to draw blood. Since beginning my rotations in the hospital, I had concocted a variety of excuses to keep from sticking needles into unlucky patients. "Oh, I have a lecture now," I'd say. Or, "I think the nurse was planning on drawing his blood," I'd lie to my resident to avoid the task at all costs. Although it worked for the most part during those first few weeks, I knew I could not escape drawing blood for long. At the end of one exhausting day, I had the second of my two encounters, this time with a middle-aged woman who—with just my luck—was deathly afraid of needles.

Outside the woman's room, one of my residents tried to teach me on the fly.

"Insert the needle with a quick, firm motion," he explained. "The quicker, the less pain, the better."

I took the advice seriously, and about two minutes later, the resident came running into the room in response to the deafening scream of my patient. Apparently, I had used too quick a movement—the needle had bounced off the woman's skin and speared her forearm about an inch away from my intended mark. She shrieked in pain while I removed the evidence. For a solid two weeks, I was the running joke of the residents. Every time I walked into their workroom, someone would make a dart-throwing motion and then burst out laughing

Not surprisingly, I'd been reluctant to try again. Tonight, however, no one else wanted to deal with the prisoner, so the duty of drawing blood had been handed down the totem pole to the lowest ranking member of the team—me. I had no choice and neither did the prisoner. My stomach churned with queasiness, and I knew that both the prisoner and I were about to have an experience that each of us would have preferred to avoid.

Under the police officer's watchful eyes, I silently went to work at the patient's bedside. Slowly I unwrapped and arranged my equipment. I tried to calm my nerves and steady my shaking hands. For my own safety and that of my family, I knew that this had to go flawlessly—no missing the vein, no causing a bruise, and no inflicting of pain.

"Your hands are shaking," the prisoner said, breaking the silence. "Are you afraid of me? Or should I be more worried that you don't know what the hell you're doing?"

"I think both," I blurted out, unable to censor my thoughts in my current state of terror.

"You've gotta relax, man," he said. "I promise I'm not going to hurt you."

For some reason, his forthrightness comforted me and I trusted him.

"Tell you what? I'll make you a deal," he said. "I'll teach you how to draw blood in return for a Snickers bar."

It seemed like a fair trade to me.

"I've had too many damn blood draws in my life for my sickle cell disease," he said, which added credibility to his case. "I could do it myself—with my eyes closed."

"It's a deal," I replied. I would have been willing to bring the man a five-course meal—a small price to avoid any future retribution for the pain I would undoubtedly cause him. Having calmed down a bit, I finished arranging the supplies and the man began his lesson.

"There, the big vein," he said. "Yeah, that one."

I tapped the inner angle of his elbow with my index finger, and his vein swelled in response. I moved to pick up the needle.

"No, no, no. Slow down," he said. "You have to hold the vein in place with one hand or you'll lose it."

I pinned his bulging vein beneath several of my fingers, and I used my other free hand to ready the needle.

"Good," he said. "Now, with steady pressure, push the needle into the vein."

I sunk the needle into his arm. He grasped the hospital blanket so tightly that his knuckles turned white. I pulled the needle out.

"I'll go get my resident," I mumbled, resigned to having botched the job once again.

"No. You're going to learn this," he ordered. "You have to hold the needle at less of an angle. If you don't, it's going to go right through the vein and into my arm—that's what you just did."

A small pocket of blood had begun to collect under the man's skin, and it reminded me of the trauma I had inflicted on my fellow medical student. Reluctantly, I opened another needle, wiped his forearm with an alcohol swab, and prepared for my next attempt.

"Aim the needle a little shallower this time."

Still shaking, I placed the needle next to his skin.

"Slow and steady pressure."

I pushed.

"Stop," he said. "There. Good."

I attached a small tube to the needle. We watched while the man's maroon blood squirted against the bottom of the vial—swirling, gathering, and miraculously filling the tube. I let out an audible sigh of relief, and my teacher smiled.

"I'll put in a good word for you," he said. "You've got the touch now."

The following morning I made a quick stop at a vending machine, and then with a Snickers bar in hand, I headed toward my patient's room. I checked with the police officer to verify whether it was okay to give the man his candy bar. The officer eyed me up and down and then shrugged. I laid the candy bar down on my teacher's tray table.

"Thanks, man," he said.

"No, thank you," I countered, feeling a bit upset that I had initially stereotyped the man as a dangerous, cold-blooded convict. Maybe he was dangerous, maybe he wasn't. Still, he'd treated me with nothing but respect. He was the first person who was patient enough to help me overcome my fear of drawing blood—an unlikely teacher, but a kind, generous, and skilled one, nonetheless.

CHAPTER FIVE

TOUCHING PEOPLE

LONG BEFORE I REACHED the entrance to his room, I could hear his ragged breathing. It sounded like the kind of panicked gasping that made me think of drowning. Indeed, he was drowning, although not in the typical sense of the word. He'd been admitted for a severe case of pneumonia—one that had filled his lungs so full of fluid that they barely had any room left for precious air.

Inside his room, I found a gaunt, disheveled man, who appeared strikingly close to my own age. He lay in a hospital bed, and he struggled to breathe through his howling oxygen mask. Slithering from beneath the scant protection of his tiny hospital gown, several gigantic reptilian tattoos crept across his shoulders, traced down his arms, and ended at his fingers. In addition, he had tattoos with the stenciled word "Jesus," several other names that I imagined belonged to his girlfriends or children, and an intimidating representation of a bull's head and horns.

"Hi, I'm Jamie," I said. I pulled up a chair next to his bed, and I made sure to give myself a few feet of space to buffer my fear. Even though I had just discharged the prisoner who had taught me why not to judge a book by its cover, as with most lessons I was learning in the hospital, it took more than a few times for things to sink in.

"Keehhvuun," he responded, conserving his words.

Sitting next to his bed, I attempted to hold a conversation with the young man—without much success. In between his raspy breaths, I collected a scattered, incoherent account of his life history, and what I heard scared me. From what I could piece together, Kevin had been involved in a gunfight several months back, which explained the wheelchair next to his bed. He belonged to a gang, which explained the gunfight. He lived on the street when he wasn't clean. And sometimes—on the rare occasion when he hadn't been drinking, or doing drugs, or both—he spent the night at his mother's house.

"Are you using drugs and sharing needles?"

"Yehhs."

"Are you having unprotected sex?"

"Yehhs."

"Are you worried about HIV and other sexually transmitted diseases?"

"Yehhs."

As I rattled off a laundry list of additional physical symptoms, Kevin nodded his head affirmatively. Unexplained weight loss? Frequent fevers? Night sweats? *Yes, yes, yes.*

I couldn't ignore Kevin's illustrious social history whether legitimate or not. Before I finished talking with him, I had already constructed a damning vision of the young man's life: he had joined a gang, gotten mixed up in sex and drugs, and—through one or both of those endeavors—acquired some transmissible disease, like HIV, that had landed him in the hospital. Although I did not have enough clinical experience (at this point I had only experienced a mere six weeks in the hospital as a medical student) to diagnose HIV from a simple social history or physical exam, I concluded that HIV was the only possible underlying cause of Kevin's pneumonia.

Nervous by the prospect of interacting with my first HIV-positive patient, my mind whirred into precautionary mode as I prepared to examine his lungs. Although I wasn't doing anything remotely invasive, like drawing blood or putting in a Foley catheter, I still plucked a pair of latex gloves from a pocket on my short white coat, and I pulled them one-by-one over each hand. As I did, the thwacking plastic-on-skin noise that filled the room caused Kevin to look up at me with an odd expression.

"I wear gloves whenever I examine a patient," I lied, and I instantly felt bad that Kevin might interpret my actions to be prejudiced. I was acting unfairly, but my fright ultimately won over my better judgment.

"Noah, yuh duunt," Kevin said, in between gasps. "Buhhhts uhhkay. I gehhht idd."

Feeling guilty, but still scared that the young man might have a communicable disease, I proceeded in silence—with my gloves on. Kevin stared straight ahead, as if to hold on to the horizon, while his body rocked from his labored breathing. If his breathing had sounded awful from a distance, his lungs sounded worse when I listened with my stethoscope. I could hear him drowning beneath the fluid contained in his chest.

A short while later, the rest of the medical team returned to Kevin's room to verify my findings. Each doctor walked out of that room with a look of amazement. Not one of us had ever found every physical sign suggestive of pneumonia in a *single* patient. Kevin had them all. The wide-eyed attending physician immediately decided to initiate treatment with high-dose antibiotics. Having already heard about Kevin's medical and social histories, and suspecting HIV as the likely culprit, the attending physician obtained consent from Kevin to perform an HIV test. Then she drew the blood herself and dropped it at the hospital lab.

Later that night, still feeling guilty about my interaction with Kevin, my mind attempted to justify my behavior. The nurse had put an intravenous line (IV) into Kevin just moments before I had met him—perhaps there could have been some contagious blood on his arm? He was disheveled and unclean—maybe he'd soiled his clothes with bodily fluids? I felt more confident about my decision to wear gloves. I had protected myself. What I'd failed to notice while I'd visited with Kevin, however, and what I realized now, was that the attending physician had touched and examined Kevin without considering using a pair of gloves. She'd just gone ahead and performed her exam.

———

Two days later, Kevin's HIV test came back—positive. Standing in front of the computer, I sucked in a deep breath. The red-flagged lab value provided confirmation that, for the first time ever (at least knowingly), I had stood in the same room with the lethal HIV virus that I'd read so much about. Oddly enough, the initial thought that crossed my mind was a selfish feeling of relief—not concern for the man, not sadness for a threatened human life, but relief that I had protected myself by treating Kevin as if he had HIV from day one. I felt exonerated from the guilty feelings that had plagued me for the past several days. "Dodged the bullet on that one," I thought.

That morning after rounds, I went back to Kevin's room with the same attending physician who had broken the bad news about cancer to Gina. Although Kevin understood that HIV was a possibility, the attending physician knew that the news would still shake him, so she allotted at least an hour to sit with Kevin and discuss his new diagnosis. On our way into Kevin's room, as had become my standard practice over the past several days, I grabbed a pair of latex gloves from the dispenser hanging next to the door. Thinking that the attending physician might want a pair too, I pocketed an extra set.

"Hi, Kevin," she said as we bustled into the room. Performing what I had learned to be her trademark maneuver, the attending physician sat in her usual position perched on the foot of the patient's bed.

"Hi, Doc," he said. He enunciated the words clearly, which signaled his drastic improvement from just days before.

"I wish I didn't have to tell you this, Kevin," she said. "That test we talked about—the one for HIV—came back positive."

He didn't flinch.

"I knew it," he said, once the initial shockwaves of fear had dissipated enough so that he could speak.

For the next thirty minutes, they continued to talk about what this new diagnosis meant for him: the different medications he could take, the various support groups he could attend, and the types of counseling he could receive. Although he exuded a surprising calm, I could still see some terror lurking behind his eyes—neither his intimidating tattoos, nor his machismo attitude could hide his fear about the possibility of death. At the end of the encounter, the attending physician stood to examine Kevin's lungs.

"I just want to take a quick listen to make sure your lungs are healing from the pneumonia."

I made a motion to hand her the extra pair of gloves, but she gave me the same look that Kevin had given me earlier: "What in the world are you thinking?" Instead, she removed her stethoscope from the pocket of her long white coat and leaned over Kevin's bed to listen to his breathing.

Honestly, I think she already knew how much better his lungs sounded and was using this opportunity as an excuse to provide Kevin with some kind of comfort. As she placed the stethoscope against his back, she used her free hand to rub his shoulder gently—the shoulder with the giant serpent tattoo creeping out from underneath his gown. If only for a moment, I swear that Kevin's entire body went slack—probably his first respite from the fright he'd experienced during the past seventy-two hours.

I felt terribly conflicted as we left the room. I wanted to emulate this attending physician, who always maintained an even hand and offered her human touch to everyone. But I still felt justified in having "protected myself" from HIV— even though I knew that it wasn't transmissible though casual contact. "You can't catch HIV from toilet seats, hugging, or even kissing," was the exact phrase that I had once used to educate college students about HIV. Nevertheless, faced with my first real HIV patient, I chose to ignore my own education. I wished I could have maintained my composure and treated Kevin with the basic dignity he deserved. In those moments after I exited Kevin's room, I couldn't shake the horrible feeling that, although I had given Kevin the medical care he required, I hadn't offered him the one thing that he probably needed most in this world: a human touch.

CHAPTER SIX

CRACKED

TOWARD THE END of my second month of the internal medicine rotation, the exhaustion of working fourteen-hour days, punctuated every fourth night by the sleepless thirty-six hours known as call, began to show in the bluish bags that hung under my eyes. More problematic than the weariness, though, my body craved some reminder of the normalcy of regular, non-hospital life. I clung to the scraps of daylight that hung in the sky while I biked home from my lengthy shifts in the hospital.

Even though standing on my feet for an entire day easily felt like more of a workout than running a marathon, some nights I still tried to jog outside along the riverside path that cut through the center of Philadelphia. Although I often plodded along at a mule's pace, the movement and fresh air rejuvenated my tired muscles and invigorated my senses.

I would jog a few miles down the river and then double back, returning to my apartment by crossing through the city's museum district. The parkway that traversed this section of town was studded with ornate wrought iron benches, which made it a popular overnight resting place for the city's homeless population.

Each day, as the last tourists left the museums and relocated downtown for dinner, the residents of the park benches would return and reclaim their territory. Before I started working at the hospital, I always ran early enough to encounter only the tourists. With my new late hours, I learned about the hidden nighttime world of the parkway, and I became acquainted with several of the more prominent inhabitants of the parkway benches.

There was a man who always wore a winter coat and other pieces of cold weather gear, despite the intolerably humid summer temperatures. On the next bench sat a woman who spewed political slander into the air, and she ranted and raved about everything from police brutality to a bomb that government agents had implanted in her uterus during a surgery. After passing several more benches, I would find my favorite of the bunch: the perpetually smiling man, whom I might have described as affable, had I not once witnessed him wearing the same smile while lunging at a group of tourists.

During one of my nightly runs, I noticed that something in the regular scenery had changed. A family of four—two parents and two small toddlers—had claimed the usually unoccupied last bench in the row. They looked new to the street, not well established like winter-coat man or perpetually smiling man. Adjacent to their bench sat two, thick garbage bags, which held the remnants of a home. Clothes spilled out of one bag, and I could see the plastic of the other bag stretched around sharp corners of picture frames. In the moments between their cautious gazes, the family shared a dinner of potato chips from a ninety-nine cent Big Grab bag and took turns swigging sips from a two-liter bottle of soda. My heart sank. I imagined the fright of sleeping on park benches with two children in tow.

By the time I made it back home, I had developed a lofty goal to help the family. But then my exhaustion from the week caught up with me, and I fell soundly asleep before I could decide how I would carry out my rescue efforts.

The following night—a call night—kept me at the hospital and provided me with my first introduction to the inside workings of the ER. The day had been surprisingly slow, and my resident had pawned me off on one of her friends working in the ER. I didn't object. I was curious to find out whether the ER lived up to the fast-paced reputation its namesake television show had created. Before I could ponder the comparison, the first patient of the night burst through a set of swinging double doors.

The man's dramatic entrance caught the ER staff by surprise. The man maniacally screamed obscenities at the top of his lungs. His wild eyes appeared to spring from his sockets, but his taut eyelids held them back. The corners of his mouth had accumulated a rabid froth. Had any people on the street witnessed his behavior, they would have instantly written the man off as a raving lunatic. Apparently in the ER, however, his behavior signaled several possibilities, the most likely of which my resident mouthed to me: "Cocaine."

By the time the man collapsed onto an empty gurney in the hallway, it was apparent that he might die. The resident and a nurse fumbled as they peeled the awkward paper backings from a tangle of sticky electrocardiogram (EKG) leads. Amazingly, they succeeded in placing the leads on the man's visibly fluttering chest. A few moments later, a series of spikes appeared on the monitor beside the gurney—not the typical blips of a heartbeat, but a chaotic mess of jagged peaks and valleys. My untrained eyes realized the EKG reading signaled that more than the man's mouth reeled out of control; the cocaine had caused his heart to beat so fast that it could barely fill with blood before exporting its precious cargo to the rest of his body.

A group of ER physicians gathered around the man's stretcher. Their forceful commands began to drown out the man's persistent commentary. Someone ordered a "push" of a medicine to slow his heart rate, and I hoped that a normal heartbeat would appear on the bedside monitor. Within a few minutes, the man's heart slowed to a reasonable pace and the EKG tracing stabilized. Even without the EKG machine, the effects of the medication were visible: his previously shuddering chest now moved peacefully in sync with his breathing. Even his mouth had quieted down.

Once the doctors had stopped the man's erratic heartbeat and replaced it with something more acceptable, the group of people assembled at the man's bedside dissipated as quickly as it had formed. The resident and I were the only ones left standing next to the man's gurney.

Knowing that the episode had secured the man an admission to the hospital, the resident didn't miss a beat. In anticipation of filling out the lengthy admission forms, she began to collect a medical history. She asked the man a series of focused questions about why he had come to the ER, if he took prescription medications, and whether he had any known medical conditions. Although he talked in short sentences, only able to string together a few words at a time before tiring, he answered each question with a surprising sincerity.

"My chest started hurting. That's why I came here. I've been here before. For the same thing. They gave me some pills last time. I ain't taken any since I ran out."

The resident pushed harder for an answer to the question that mattered.

"Why did your chest start hurting? Were you using any drugs at the time?"

The candid answer that followed startled me more than the frantic blitz of medical intervention I had just witnessed.

"Mmmm. Yeah, my brother and me. We was smokin' some crack. Shit, I'm gettin' too old for this."

"How many days in the last week have you smoked?"

"Every day."

The resident proceeded to collect as much additional background information as she could, but the man soon dozed off mid-sentence. Nevertheless, she had gathered the facts that she needed to arrange a bed for the man in the cardiac ward. We retreated to the nurses' station to begin the admission process.

Even though the ER admits patients to the hospital all night long, the remainder of the hospital still follows a nine-to-five schedule. This means that an overnight skeleton team of physicians stabilized most patients, and then they waited until the following morning, once the rest of the medical team was present, to discuss, debate, and decide on a course of treatment. Accordingly, we spent the remainder of the night ironing out the details of the patient's admission and preparing for rounds the following morning. I also tackled what I had learned to be a designated job of the medical student: tracking down and reviewing the several inches of paper that made up a patient's medical record.

Fortunately, I had visited the medical record office numerous times during the previous three weeks, and although I still couldn't find the cafeteria without getting lost, on this particular night I stumbled upon the correct door. I rang a small bell on a desk and a woman appeared in the window. I wondered whether she ever left the tiny, cramped nook carved out from the overstuffed shelves of patient charts.

"Patient name?"

"Alden Dowd."

She turned on her heels and disappeared, swallowed up by the cavernous rows of medical records. Just a few minutes later, she reappeared with the thickest medical chart I had ever seen and hefted it onto the counter.

"You have fun with that one, honey," she said, and then she was gone.

Back in the ER, I sat at the nurses' station and purposefully read each page of Alden's medical record. He'd been to the ER a half-dozen times in the last year, and he had been admitted to the hospital on several of those occasions, each time with complaints of chest pain. During one of the previous visits, his physicians had diagnosed him with congestive heart failure (CHF) secondary to several old heart attacks, and they had started him on pills that made him pee out the extra water in his body. Follow-up appointments had been made and free bottles of medication had been given. Nevertheless, judging by the number of past hospitalizations for the same exact problem, Alden wasn't doing a good job of taking care of himself. Especially in light of his earlier comment: "Every day."

Even though doctors—and by extension, medical students— are supposed to treat all patients with an even hand, my composure cracked. I became fiercely angry with Alden. The heft of his chart suggested he had ignored hundreds and thousands of dollars worth of medical care, and my anger intensified after remembering the family in the park.

Whether I could justifiably compare the two situations, I imagined how much of a difference just a fraction of the money spent on Alden's care would have made to that struggling family. Deciding I would grapple with it later so that maybe I could get some sleep that night, I wearily continued with my review of his thick chart.

CHAPTER SEVEN

AGAINST MEDICAL ADVICE

"**Y**OU'RE ON," MY SUPERVISING RESIDENT mouthed to me.

The previous night, she had decided to have me present Alden Dowd's case during "Bedside Rounds." Once a week, the medical team picked a day to visit the bedside of one or two interesting or complicated patients. While standing beside the patient, the medical student or resident would present the patient's medical history, and then the entire medical team would examine the patient. Since I was "on," I would have to strike a most intimidating balance in my delivery of Alden's story: respectfully presenting his personal history—drugs, sex, and alcohol—while faithfully reviewing the pertinent aspects of his medical history. I knew I would have to choose my words carefully to avoid criticism from Alden, the attending physician, or both. Somehow, I figured, I'd mess it up. Still, I was too angry with Alden to care about what he thought of me.

After we gathered around Alden's bedside, I told his story. I tactfully tried to present that he was noncompliant with all aspects of his medical care, despite his physician's multiple attempts to ensure regular follow-up care. "Noncompliant" was the nice, politically correct word for "careless," and secretly

I hoped that Alden didn't understand what I had implied. He didn't flinch, so I continued, and I wondered whether he would raise an eyebrow when I mentioned his cocaine habit. Although I would have chosen to talk about the issue in an entirely different setting—one without Alden sitting next to me—I took a deep breath and gave it my best shot.

"Alden lives with his brother in an apartment in the city. He is unemployed, so his younger brother supports the two of them by dealing drugs. Every so often, Alden uses crack cocaine. He reports that in the last week, he has used it more frequently than usual. He denies using any drugs other than cocaine."

I watched Alden's eyes carefully, but he wasn't startled or angered by my comments. Much like the previous night, it surprised me that he acknowledged his drug habit so matter-of-factly. From everything I had learned, both in college and in medical school, people with addictions *never* gave in that easily. Nevertheless, I appreciated his honesty, and more a reflection of my naïveté than anything else, his forthrightness continued to impress me.

His candor, however, did not fool the rest of the team. Once we exited the room, the attending physician outlined her recommendations: "Order a cardiology consult, restart his CHF medications, draw labs, and get a urine drug screen."

I wondered why in the world we needed a drug screen. He had admitted openly to using cocaine! After the attending physician finished giving her instructions, I sheepishly spoke up.

"Don't we already know that he's taking drugs? Why do we need to get a drug screen?"

She merely responded, "Why do you think?"

She was correct to order the screen. The toxicology panel came back that afternoon with three, red-flagged lab values: heroin, amphetamines, and marijuana. Alden was a walking medicine cabinet, but his body wasn't filled with his prescribed blood pressure medications. Instead, Alden's blood coursed with multiple, illegal substances. The results of the drug screen angered me more—I felt partly upset that he lied to me and partly upset that I had believed him. But more disturbing was my sudden insight into why the heft of Alden's medical chart had bothered me so much: making an impact on this man's life would require more cooperation from him than he was probably capable of giving.

During the next several days, Alden underwent multiple tests that confirmed the poor condition of his heart. He suffered from severely uncontrolled CHF, although this time, the doctors remained suspicious that the cocaine had irreversibly damaged his heart. To evaluate this, Alden needed to undergo cardiac catheterization—an expensive, risky operative procedure that provides precise measurements regarding a heart's function.

Indeed, compared to the studies performed during his previous visits, the catheterization revealed that Alden's heart had lost a significant amount of function. Once the team had discussed the study results, the attending physician sat down with Alden. She explained that if he had another episode like the one in the ER, he would die. Alden needed to quit his cocaine habit—immediately.

Alden agreed with a vigorous nod.

"Yes, Doc. I know. I'm done with crack."

Much to my delight, Alden's health and attitude underwent a drastic change. The information from the cardiac catheterization allowed the medical team to titrate Alden's heart medications to their optimal dosages. As his medications built up to therapeutic levels, Alden's general appearance improved commensurately.

He felt better, too. In the mornings, Alden would strike up a conversation.

"I saw an infomercial last night on the Jack LaLanne Juice-O-Matic—I have to get me one of those." Or he would talk about what he had for dinner the previous night and how much he had enjoyed it. For those first several days after Alden started to feel better, he displayed the characteristics of a model patient:

someone working happily and diligently toward the sole goal of improving his life.

After three or four days of steady improvement, it stunned me when Alden's attitude took a sudden and dramatic turn for the worse. One morning as I entered his room, expecting to hear the wonders of the Jack LaLanne Juice-O-Matic or the benefits of amazing OxiClean powder, I was greeted instead by silent, seething rage.

Alden refused to look at or speak to me. He fixed his gaze on some imaginary speck on the wall as if I did not exist. I noticed that the vein coursing across his temple bulged and throbbed and that it served as a small, external thermometer of his internal fury. His breathing was also markedly labored, and he struggled to take each breath—significantly more than he had the last several days. He wouldn't talk to me, so I finished my physical exam and left the room.

The attending physician, who happened to be in the hallway outside Alden's room, saw the concerned look on my face.

"Remember this. It's classic," she said. "After a few days of feeling better on the right medications, how quickly he forgets how crappy he felt a few days ago. I'm sure Alden's craving to get high right now, especially since we've just proven to him that we can treat him with medicines when something goes wrong. What he doesn't realize is that we won't always be able to fix him. He's lucky this time. But if he continues to use more cocaine or amphetamines, he can kiss his heart good-bye. We can't save dead muscle."

I peered through the small window in Alden's door and watched him talk irately into the receiver of his phone. I couldn't hear his obviously furious monologue, but I could tell the conversation was not about some infomercial product. If the attending physician was correct, the conversation was about a different kind of product.

With each passing day, Alden's disgust at the medical staff grew exponentially. His fuming morning silences progressed to unrestrained shouting sessions each time the medical team entered his room.

"Stop poisoning me, you ignorant fools," he said. He would sputter and spit, his eyes wild, and his hands furiously emphasizing his words. "You're conspiring to keep me here against my will!"

In actuality, the resident and I had spent a significant amount of time working on his discharge plans. We secured a rehabilitation bed despite his lack of insurance, spent hours on the phone with the city health department to ensure he would receive his heart medications at no charge, and located information about subsidized housing for indigent seniors.

Nevertheless, Alden's dissatisfaction escalated to a point where our team could do nothing to pacify him. During rounds the next morning, when the team entered Alden's room, he sat bolt upright, yanked the sticky EKG leads off his chest, and swore under his breath.

"I've had enough of this shit," he said, and then he climbed out of his bed.

While the attending physician verbally attempted to soothe him, Alden dialed a number on the phone, and then he angrily instructed his brother to come to the hospital immediately. He slammed the receiver back into its cradle and leered at the attending physician.

"Where's my paper to sign? I'm outta here!"

The attending physician began to explain what signing out against medical advice (AMA) meant.

"Speaking as your doctor, I don't think you are well enough to leave the hospital yet," she said. "I'd recommend that you stay put."

"Don't you threaten me, bitch! Gimme that paper," Alden responded.

A few minutes later, after Alden had scrawled his name across the bottom of an AMA form (which, to my surprise, were used so frequently that the forms were pre-printed), he continued to dress himself and gather his belongings. He paused in front of his small bathroom mirror, combed his hair back into a slick mane, and then slapped on his thick, black-rimmed sunglasses. After picking up his small leather bag, he turned on his heels and walked right past the medical team and out of his hospital room.

Alden tossed me a cool glance from behind his dark-tinted lenses, but I couldn't tell whether his eyes held spite, or thanks, or indifference. I watched him strut silently down the hallway and swagger through the swinging double doors of the ER toward his brother's idling station wagon. The passenger side door kicked open, Alden got in, and the last memory I have of him was an old car coughing out a cloud of soot as it sped away.

That night I ran along the river to ease some of my frustration with the entire ordeal. As usual, I plodded toward the parkway benches—but this time, I carried oranges, bananas, and two candy bars in my small backpack. I decided I would feed the homeless family. I needed to feel like I could make a small, positive difference to counteract the medical team's negative experience with Alden.

I ran past the man with beaded sweat running down his face, past the woman yelling, "I'm gonna explode if you come any nearer," past the man with the maniacal smile, and that's where I found the empty bench usually occupied by the family. I felt somewhat relieved to imagine that they had found their way to a shelter, or maybe returned to their home. The feeling of relief disappeared the moment I spied the telltale bulges of their bags peeking from behind the bench. I laid the contents of my knapsack on the bench, and then I hurried back toward my apartment.

I decided I couldn't compare the family's situation with the hundreds of thousands of dollars wasted on Alden's medical care. I knew—and believed—that a physician was supposed to be impartial, to treat everyone with unyielding fairness and without discrimination, but I still couldn't help from imagining how many bananas and oranges the money spent on one cardiac catheterization might have bought—not to mention how many months of rent it could have paid for the homeless family.

I didn't yet know how to remain impartial when a patient like Alden walked out of one door and into another—not the door of another hospital or rehabilitation center, but through the door of his usual haunt: a crack house. I imagined he'd be coming back through the ER doors in a few days or weeks, maybe alive or maybe dead, and I wasn't sure he'd care either way. In the meantime, the nights grew colder, and the kids missed another week of school.

CHAPTER EIGHT

WITHOUT QUESTION

"LISTEN, I'M RUNNING BEHIND. The patient in the last room hurt his knee yesterday. Go in, introduce yourself, and give your best shot at performing a knee exam. Find me when you're done."

Earlier that week, after three months of working in the inpatient medicine ward, I had happily traded life in the hospital to work with a family doctor who ran a solo practice in a nearby town. For the next month, I would assist Dr. Freedman and see the other side of medicine—the side that was easy to lose track of while in the high-stakes environment of the hospital. Now I would learn about things like how to manage high blood pressure, titrate up cholesterol medications, counsel on the benefits of smoking cessation, perform knee and back exams for sciatica—the meat and potatoes stuff of doctoring.

Even though my classmates had warned me about how mind-numbing office practice could be, I looked forward to the break from the long shifts in the hospital. I figured I could temporarily forgo learning about the management of complex and rare diseases in exchange for a month of easier days and no overnight calls—even if it meant doing bland, routine things like writing script after script after script for blood pressure medications.

While the initial several days had been interesting enough, by the end of the first week I was officially bored by outpatient medicine. I didn't have the experience to make that kind of claim—at this stage of my training, every experience had the potential to be educational. Yet, knowing that most visits would end with Dr. Freedman either writing a prescription refill for a blood pressure medicine or sending the patient off to a specialist for further evaluation of an interesting problem, I found myself shutting off the creative, analytic side of my mind before I entered a patient's room.

For the patient who needed the knee exam, I had already decided that either Dr. Freedman would send him home to take ibuprofen and ice his knee, or he would refer him to a sports medicine doctor for a more extensive work-up. In either case, the patient required little additional thought on my part.

After I picked up George Levy's patient chart, I walked down the hall and ducked my head into the tiny examining room to see whether Mr. Levy had donned a hospital gown. He had not.

"Would you mind putting on this gown? And then I'll come back to examine you." I thrust a paper gown through the crack in the door.

Mr. Levy hesitated, and as I peeked into the exam room, I could see a quizzical look on his face. He stood, walked comfortably across the small room, and grabbed the small gown from my extended hand.

"Sure. You need me to undress, Doc?"

"Yes," I said.

A few minutes later, I returned to the small room and began the examination. I bent, pulled, pried, and twisted Mr. Levy's leg, trying to re-create the maneuvers depicted in my physical exam atlas. No matter how faithfully I performed the various exercises, I could not elicit any pain. If he had actually hurt his anterior cruciate ligament (a common type of knee injury), then I should have at least been able to provoke a bit of discomfort. I repeated each maneuver twice, and by the end of the procedure,

I felt certain that the man had not truly injured his knee. Ice and ibuprofen it was—another less-than-interesting case.

"I think your knee is okay."

"I know," Mr. Levy said as he rolled his eyes at me. Although this should have set off a warning bell in my head, in my attempt to be efficient, I began to scribble the results of my exam on a blank page in Mr. Levy's chart.

"Dr. Freedman will be in shortly to check for himself. As long as he doesn't find anything of concern, you'll need to take some ibuprofen for a few days, ice your knee, and give yourself a bit of rest."

"Whatever you say."

Back in the hallway, as I kept watch for Dr. Freedman, I pre-wrote a script for ibuprofen that Dr. Freedman could sign, so that we could get the patient on his way. Dr. Freedman finished with another patient, and then he hurriedly directed me toward the room of my patient. While we walked down the hall, he explained that because of the chaotic schedule, he would do the talking and I could present my own findings later.

"How are you?" he asked Mr. Levy as we entered the examination room. They shook hands, and as Dr. Freedman saw his gowned patient, a peculiar look crossed his face.

"George, I thought we only needed to talk about your blood pressure medications today. It's not already time for your annual physical, is it?"

"Nope, I'm just here for more water pills."

The moment I heard those words, my stomach turned upside down. Dr. Freedman had specifically asked me to perform a knee exam on this patient, but why a knee exam if the man only needed adjustment of his medications? I stood bewildered in the corner while Dr. Freedman and Mr. Levy finished their discussion about the man's diuretics. As we began to leave the room to let Mr. Levy dress, he stammered a moment.

"Doc … um … is something wrong with my knee?"

"No, not at all," Dr. Freedman responded, matter-of-factly.

"Oh. Well, good then."

Later that afternoon, once things had calmed down, Dr. Freedman slyly asked me how my "knee exam" had gone.

"Uh, fine, I think," I said. Still uncertain about what had occurred earlier, I felt my face flush.

With a chuckle, Dr. Freedman then explained that his nurse had switched the rooms of his two eleven o'clock patients. The person with the injured knee had been unable to walk down the hall, so the nurse had put him in the nearest exam room. I had seen the other patient—the one without a knee problem, the one who only needed his blood pressure medications refilled.

"I just like to keep you on your toes," Dr. Freedman said. "I know how easy it can be to get lost in the routine of things."

While Dr. Freedman seemed amused by my mistake, the experience thoroughly shook me up. This time my blunder meant that a man had unnecessarily endured the temporary humiliation of wearing a revealing hospital gown and the discomfort of my twisting, prodding hands—I could come to terms with that. But what was more difficult to accept was what *could* have happened. What if I had been the one in charge and the procedure was not as innocent as a simple knee exam? Suppose I ordered an incorrect medication or an unnecessary test for the wrong patient.

In the office later that afternoon, before I saw each of the remaining patients, I took a few extra seconds and reminded myself to stop, look up for a moment, and make sure that I performed a knee exam on someone who actually had knee pain.

CHAPTER NINE

HOME

"**A**RE YOU HERE TO FIX the refrigerator?" asked a woman sitting in a wheelchair beside the nurses' station.

"No," I replied. "I'm helping Dr. Freedman today."

"What?" she said, a bit louder this time. "The refrigerator is that way!" She pointed down the hallway.

Figuring she was a bit deaf, I tried once more, this time speaking at the top of my lungs, to convince her that I was not a Maytag repairman.

"No, I am here to help Dr. Freedman."

"Oh, the doctor? Yes, he'll pay you after you fix the refrigerator."

Dr. Freedman motioned for me, smiling as I approached.

"I see you've met Rita. She's just about the sweetest woman in the world. But be prepared—she'll create a new identity for you each time you meet her."

Every other afternoon, Dr. Freedman closed his office for two hours so we could see patients at a local nursing home where he served as the medical director. Each day we would round on six or seven patients so that by the end of the week, we had visited everyone in the fifteen-bed nursing home and updated their orders for the coming week.

Earl was an eighty-year-old World War II veteran with mild Alzheimer's disease, as well as a history of poorly controlled diabetes. Earl's family members, claiming his presence was the equivalent of "having another teenager in the house," were unable to care for him any longer, and they placed him in a nursing home.

Earl did have a reckless streak. The previous evening, he had escaped from the nursing home by sneaking out of the locked unit and walking along a major highway to a local bar. There he met his girlfriend. She had refused to visit him in the nursing home out of fear they would keep her there, too. Like Earl, she had the beginnings of Alzheimer's disease, but her condition was complicated by mild paranoia.

Before Earl could get a word out, Dr. Freedman, although thirty years Earl's junior, took the strong position of a disappointed father.

"Earl, you can't just leave the unit. Especially not to go to a bar! The police brought you back drunk. Your blood sugars were through the roof!"

"But I wanted to show my girl a good time," Earl said.

Dr. Freedman paused a moment while he suppressed a smile, and then, regaining his composure and resuming a frown, he patiently continued to reason with Earl.

"I know you wanted to see your girlfriend, Earl, but there are safer ways to do it. She can come here to visit you. That's not a problem."

"No hot babe is gonna want to date a geezer stuck in an old folks home. I've got a reputation to maintain."

"I promise we'll stay out of your hair if she wants to visit you here. You can have your privacy. I just don't want to have to call the police again. You scared us all when you disappeared."

"You know how to wreck an old man's fun," Earl muttered.

"I'm sorry, Earl," said Dr. Freedman. "Honestly, I am. But I promise that I will work with you so you can have the independence you're used to. Try to remember that I'm looking out for your safety because I care about you, Earl. I don't want to see anything bad happen to you."

Like a disgruntled teenager, Earl ignored Dr. Freedman's concerned remarks, and he turned up the volume of his blaring television. He didn't say another word while we finished examining him.

After we left the room, Dr. Freedman burst out laughing.

"And here I thought that I was done dealing with teenagers," he said, grinning. "I just sent my youngest son off to college, and here we go all over again!"

Then, in a slightly lower voice, he continued. "As funny as it seems, I hate being put in that position. It's the worst part of this job. Here's a man who's lived his whole life independently. Now he lives according to a schedule of story groups, meals, and exercises. Even his JELL-O snack is delivered at the same time every day. He wants to see his girlfriend, he wants to have a beer occasionally, and I don't blame him. I wish I could let him. But I'm put in the awkward fatherly role, and I have to be incredibly strict so I don't get sued."

With that, the smile returned, and he finished by echoing Earl's own words, "I've got a reputation to maintain."

"The devil will not prevail! The devil will not prevail!" screeched Attie, from farther down the hallway. I was surprised to find a tiny, frail woman with a deceivingly intimidating voice.

"Hi, Attie," said Dr. Freedman.

As we entered the room, Attie's visitor wheeled herself out of the room, calling behind her, "Thanks, Attie!"

"And don't ever forget," Attie boomed from behind, "that you will rise above all of this."

Dr. Freedman had tried to prepare me for this by giving me some background information about Attie: She had been the wife of a community minister. Since her husband died several years earlier, Attie had assumed his role, at first in the community, but more recently within the nursing home. She held a daily prayer session for her small congregation of nursing home residents, and a few times per week, she held confessionals, similar to the one we had just interrupted.

Several days earlier, Dr. Freedman had contacted Attie's children to arrange a family meeting to discuss Attie's do not resuscitate (DNR) status. Although Attie had remained in stable health—the best one could wish for at the age of ninety-seven—Dr. Freedman was still concerned that her condition could change for the worse at any moment.

Attie had a history of valvular heart disease that could cause flash pulmonary edema—her lungs could fill up with fluid. If the edema occurred again, it would leave Attie in a tenuous state of health. Dr. Freedman firmly believed in being prepared. As he did with all of his patients, he wanted to discuss the goals and limitations of Attie's care, so he could ensure that the last days of her life would be in concert with how she had lived her earlier years. So, at Attie's request, he invited her family to join the discussion.

After spending five minutes greeting the half-dozen children and grandchildren who had shown up for the family meeting, Dr. Freedman began.

"Attie, as you know, we are all here because each one of us wants to make sure that you continue to live your life in the way that you want."

Attie, never one to hold back, interrupted.

"Let's get right down to it, sweetie. When the Lord decides that my time has come, it is he who will decide, not me. I've been blessed for the last ninety-seven years and each extra day that I get is nothing short of a miracle."

Her children, aware of their mother's steadfast beliefs, nodded. Still, everyone wanted to know the specifics of what she intended. Her oldest child spoke up to inquire about what kinds of things Attie might like done if she had another episode of pulmonary edema, or suffered from some other debilitating insult. Would she want food? Antibiotics for treatable infections? Pain medication?

Attie remained firm and clear in her wishes. "It's out of my hands, and it's out of your hands, too. When God decides to take me, that's when I will go from this world. I don't want you to do anything to keep me from joining him in heaven."

While everyone was considering her reply, a voice called from outside the door.

"Attie, you ready for me yet?" A small, frail elderly resident rolled her wheelchair partway into the room before realizing that we were in the middle of a private conversation.

"Oh, I'm sorry," she said, trying to back her wheelchair up.

"No, no, dear. Come on in, we were just finishing," Attie replied. Then, addressing the rest of us, she said, "Now if you will excuse me, I have appointments scheduled all afternoon."

Her family members smiled, as did Dr. Freedman, and everyone shuffled out of the room so Attie could continue advising her congregants about living a fulfilling life.

After leaving Attie and her children behind, we reached the room of our final patient of the day: Ryan, a twenty-year-old who'd been paralyzed from the neck down in his late teens following a dirt biking accident. Ryan ended up in the nursing home after his family had exhausted their physical, mental, and monetary resources trying to care for him at home—that was how Dr. Freedman had nicely camouflaged it, but I could sense from his explanation that Ryan had grown up in an unstable living environment. From down the hallway, I could see Ryan perched in his wheelchair. His face lit up as soon as he saw us coming, and Dr. Freedman, whom up until this point I had only known as a conservative man, said, "Hey, dude! What's hanging?"

53

"Not much," Ryan responded with a smile. "Who's your friend?"

"This is Jamie," said Dr. Freedman. "He's a medical student who's helping me out for a few weeks."

I sheepishly waved a silent hello. I felt like an intruder on a conversation between two old friends. Then, already feeling awkward, I wondered whether I had just insulted Ryan: I hadn't considered that he couldn't wave back. Stupid, stupid, stupid—I should have just said hello. But Ryan didn't seem to think anything more of it. His thoughts turned to the Super Bowl.

"Hey, Dr. Freedman," Ryan said. "Did you catch the game yesterday?"

"Nope. I was at the office catching up on my charts."

"How do you miss the Super Bowl?" Ryan responded, playfully prodding Dr. Freedman. "Nothing's that important!"

Dr. Freedman chuckled.

Ryan, knowing the routine, used a mouth-controlled joystick to motor his wheelchair back into his room. He spent half his day in the chair and half his day in his bed, which had a similarly futuristic contraption that shifted him from side to side to avoid putting too much pressure on any one patch of his skin. For immobile patients, preventing skin breakdown often became a difficult medical problem to manage, especially in a large patient like Ryan. Looking at his big-boned frame, I thought that Ryan must have been a gigantic human before his accident, when he actually had some meat on his bones. Still, the weight of his atrophied body was enough to cause significant pressure sores and skin breakdown. Dr. Freedman had told me to prepare myself for the stench of Ryan's open wounds.

Then Dr. Freedman and I—two scrawny, bookish men in shirts and ties—hoisted Ryan out of his wheelchair and into his hospital bed. Dr. Freedman rolled Ryan to his side so that we could examine the skin around Ryan's buttocks. The tissue there had become red and inflamed, and in places, the skin no longer protected the inside from the outside. The stench was unbearable, but Dr. Freedman didn't wince at the putrid air. He changed the dressing, chatted with Ryan the entire time about football, and then rolled Ryan back over to talk to him face-to-face.

"Ryan, I know you don't want to go back to the hospital. But I think they are going to need to clean out the dead tissue around your wound. You might need a skin graft, too," Dr. Freedman said. "The last thing I want is for that wound to become infected."

In a nonchalant manner, Ryan agreed. He seemed to trust Dr. Freedman implicitly—Dr. Freedman's word was all he needed. Then Ryan returned the conversation to sports, and within a few moments, he and Dr. Freedman were back to their playful, joking selves. It was clear that the best part of Ryan's day was when he connected with someone about something other than an aberrant lab value, or his appetite, or how many bowel movements he'd had in the previous twenty-four hours.

Even though Dr. Freedman's main responsibility was to worry about Ryan's medical care, I could sense that his companionship provided Ryan with something just as beneficial. While talking to Dr. Freedman, Ryan had the carefree look of someone whose most serious concern was that his favorite team had just lost the Super Bowl.

"Hey, good-lookin'!" Rita called at me, already forgetting that moments earlier she had mistaken me for a Maytag repairman. "You must be a movie star with those handsome eyes. Tell me, which films have I seen you in?"

"I'm just here with Dr. Freedman, Rita," I said, somewhat reluctant to give up my new movie star status. "I'm practicing to become a doctor."

"Oh, I see. You're researching your new part."

Although I did not live up to the various roles that Rita created for me, the more I thought about it, the more I realized that Dr. Freedman probably did. Of course, he really wasn't a Maytag man or a movie star, but he did wear many different guises while working in the nursing home. Here, at this intersection between the lives of Dr. Freedman and his patients, I discovered where Dr. Freedman practiced his true medicine. In his office, I had seen only snapshots of Dr. Freedman's longstanding histories with his patients—I witnessed just one or two visits out of the hundreds or thousands that he would share with his patients during the courses of their lives. I had mistakenly concluded that primary care medicine couldn't possibly hold a candle to the fast pace and intrigue of hospital medicine. The lab tests, the cholesterol checks, the adjustment of blood pressure medications—these were all undoubtedly important aspects of Dr. Freedman's job, but as he openly admitted to me, they were not necessarily the most stimulating. Yet, once I looked beyond these things, once I realized the depth of the relationships that Dr. Freedman had formed with his patients, I stood in awe of what he did for each of his patients and their families.

"I'll see you on the movie screen, sweetie!" Rita called from behind me as Dr. Freedman and I left the nursing home that afternoon. I chuckled as I waved good-bye. She didn't realize that the real star of the show was walking beside me, the corners of his mouth just barely forming a humble smile.

Chapter Ten

Bag of Humility

A FTER DR. FREEDMAN PARKED next to the weathered mailbox, and we climbed out of his dilapidated car, I saw Jack standing in his garage. Surrounded by years of accumulated boots, sleds, and rusted bikes, he looked lost. It was my final day with Dr. Freedman, and fittingly, we were making a house call to see a woman I had met during my first week of work in Dr. Freedman's office. The patient's husband, Jack, greeted us with a firm handshake, and then he started in about how he needed new shelves to organize the clutter.

"Sorry it's such a mess. I meant to pick up before you came. But Hannah needed some company this morning."

As he had the first time I met him at the office, Jack continued to talk about his garden and his other new projects— some of his old ones, too—chatting away as if he hadn't seen Dr. Freedman in years. After we navigated to the back of the garage, we passed through a thick wooden doorframe into a dark hallway.

"Don't worry about taking off your shoes. You can go back and visit with Hannah. I'll get some refreshments together. How about some vegetables from the garden?" Jack said, and then disappeared into the kitchen.

Still out in the hallway, I noticed that the worn pathways in the shag carpet revealed the couple's favorite rooms. Off to the left, the family den had walls filled with trinkets and pictures, and there was a bunny-eared television in the corner. Off to the right, the tiny kitchen where Jack stood contained a small table filled with Monday-to-Sunday pillboxes and a stack of old mail. Straight ahead, the bedroom, their once quiet retreat, had now turned into the center of their world. Hannah sat upright in a recliner next to their bed. Her head slumped against her left shoulder.

Dr. Freedman told me that he'd known Jack and Hannah since he had begun practicing in the area nearly ten years ago. Dr. Freedman also took care of their three sons, a handful of their grandchildren, and a number of their other relatives. He knew the family well, and he knew that Hannah stood at the center of their world. Her son had confided in us several days earlier at the office that his mother wasn't doing well, but neither of us realized just how much Hannah's health had deteriorated.

A month earlier, when I met Jack and Hannah for the first time, Hannah's main worry was her hoarse voice. Dr. Freedman had ordered a chest radiograph to investigate the cause. Two days later, he called the couple back into the office to let them know that the radiograph had revealed a large lung tumor. Hannah took the news with surprising resolve—she bit her lower lip, almost as if she expected the diagnosis. Jack sat stunned and silent beside her. He held her hand and ever so slightly rubbed his thumb across the back of it.

"Docs, would you like a cucumber? Here, help yourselves," Jack said. His voice brought me back to the current moment. He had finished in the kitchen, and as he hobbled into the bedroom, he set down a plate of sliced cucumbers and peppers. Jack rattled on about his latest hobby of weaving wicker baskets, while he moved behind Hannah to place his hands on her shoulders and gently massage them.

Dr. Freedman knelt in front of Hannah on the raggedy carpet. As he opened his black leather bag to take out his stethoscope, an overwhelming sadness enveloped me. The strong woman sat wilted in her chair. She had a painfully empty stare.

After Dr. Freedman finished, he handed me the stethoscope. I barely heard Hannah's heartbeat over my thumping pulse or her respirations over my anxious breaths. But before taking her vital signs, I knew Hannah would die soon. Still, I clutched to my normal routine out of fear of otherwise losing myself to heavy sorrow. As I watched Dr. Freedman press his hands against her abdomen and feel the fluid in her swollen legs, I could only think of Jack sitting alone at the kitchen table without anyone to listen to his ideas.

While we finished examining Hannah, I noticed that Jack was rubbing Hannah's shoulder almost without moving his fingers— the same way he had in Dr. Freedman's office several months earlier. I imagined it was the most tender movement Jack's coarse laborer's hand had ever made, and somehow I immediately knew that Jack understood Hannah didn't have much time left. I stared in amazement—Jack placed the love of fifty years of marriage in a protective touch, as if to shield his wife from the hurtful truth.

Dr. Freedman began to muster the strength to speak, but before he could, Jack motioned toward the kitchen.

"Why don't we go eat in the other room? Hannah seems tired," he said. He would show us his latest recipes, too. Then Jack nodded his wrinkled brow toward the hallway and ushered us out of the room.

By the time we reached the kitchen, Dr. Freedman still had no words to address Hannah's approaching fate. He made a number of meandering attempts to talk with Jack, but as if anticipating Dr. Freedman's intentions, Jack shifted the topic of conversation each time.

"Our oldest just got a promotion," he said. "Our grand-daughter just learned to walk."

Although both of us understood what Jack was trying to do, Dr. Freedman felt obliged to talk with him before we left. In lieu of words, Dr. Freedman took out his script pad and wrote a prescription for pain medicine.

"Here, this will ease her pain during these last few days," Dr. Freedman explained.

Although Jack's shaky hand accepted the prescription, his words would not betray his intent. He continued to pull out tattered recipes from cardboard containers, and he handed the most worn ones to Dr. Freedman.

"That's Hannah's favorite—I've got string beans in the garden to make it with."

After we sat and talked about everything except Hannah, we rose to leave.

"Hold on a moment," Jack said. He'd just picked some lettuce and wanted Dr. Freedman to take some.

With a plastic bag of lettuce in one hand and his black physician's bag in the other, Dr. Freedman and I followed Jack as he shuffled down the hallway toward the door. After we descended the stairs into the garage, Jack placed his thick hand on Dr. Freedman's shoulder.

"You'll come to the funeral?"

Dr. Freedman nodded, and I could see his body visibly relax as if a huge weight had just been lifted from his shoulders. We then walked back down the driveway while Jack stood in the same place where we initially found him. He waved good-bye, and then disappeared into the house as we drove away.

Balancing the little bag of lettuce on my lap, I silently reflected on the humility of Jack's gift. It was simple and human, much like what I had felt today in their home. At that moment, despite all of the second-guessing I had done during the past several months about my decision to enter medical school, I felt that I had made the right choice to enter this profession. No doubt, I still had much to learn and many years of training ahead, but I imagined myself caring for people in the way that Dr. Freedman did—there was nothing I wanted to do more.

OBSTETRICS & GYNECOLOGY

CHAPTER ELEVEN

NO INSTRUCTIONS REQUIRED

J UST WHEN I WAS GETTING the hang of surviving in the field of internal medicine, the rotation ended. Now, I was scheduled to broaden my medical education by learning about obstetrics and gynecology (OB-GYN)—two subjects I knew *nothing* about. To be truthful, I wasn't sure I wanted to know anything about either one. In that all-too-familiar way, I felt as if the rug had been pulled from underneath me and I was being thrust into another foreign situation. I'd have to adopt a completely different way of thinking about things—this time through the eyes of an obstetrician or a gynecologist. Of course, I would also have to discover all the preferences, customs, and quirks of the hospital's labor and delivery ward—a place I had not visited since I'd been born.

I reported early the following Monday morning for my orientation to the OB-GYN clerkship. The course director assigned each medical student to one of the several available combinations of labor and delivery, outpatient clinic, and gynecologic surgery. I started on the labor and delivery ward. Despite my trepidation associated with starting a new rotation, I was thrilled to know that I would get to witness the childbirth process—something that, for a long time, I had expected would be the crowning moment of my medical school experience.

No sooner had I arrived at the residents' lounge on the labor and delivery floor, than we were off and running down the hallway in response to a piercing, bloodcurdling scream.

"Uughhh! Shhhhhhhhhit. Owwwww!"

If we had been standing on a public street corner, I might have expected to see someone lying murdered in a pool of blood—the scream was that horrifying. But, we weren't standing on a street corner, and I realized I was about to witness my first birth, and by the sounds of it, soon.

I followed my new supervising resident into a small anteroom where she gave me a three-sentence crash course on the mechanics of delivering a baby.

"Stand and catch the baby. Don't drop it. That's about all there is to it."

I followed her lead as she dressed herself in a plastic gown, knee-high paper booties, and a plastic face shield. By the end of the process, I wondered why we were dressed like astronauts. Were they sending me in to practice delivering some nonhuman life form before I could attempt to help any real human patients? Maybe that explained the strange screams coming from the adjoining room.

We entered the room where the patient lay, and I realized that a living human being was making the sounds. At the head of the bed, a young man stood dressed in a costume similar to mine. He smoothed back several strands of hair that had fallen loose from behind the shrieking, pregnant woman's ear. He had the same terrified expression that I imagined was plastered across my own face.

One of the other residents had already perched herself between the pregnant woman's spread knees. Every few moments, when the expectant mother paused from her screaming long enough to suck in a deep breath, the resident would take advantage of the opportunity and offer a few words of encouragement.

"Good, push a little longer! Yes, that's perfect! Relax and breathe."

From behind me, I felt someone nudging me forward, and then I recognized the supervising resident's voice as she whispered in my ear.

"This one's yours."

Once I understood what she meant, my stomach turned inside out. I thought, "No, you must be mistaken. I am just supposed to stand here and watch. This is my first day. I've never even held a baby!"

The other resident, sensing my presence and knowing better than I the role of a medical student, quickly introduced me to the screaming patient.

"Barbara, this is—" the resident said, realizing she didn't know my name. Then, she turned to face me. "What's your name?"

"Jamie."

"Barbara, this is Jamie. He's going to help me deliver your baby."

"Uughhh! I don't caaaaaare. Just get this thing out of me. Now!"

The resident grabbed my gloved hand and placed it underneath her own. I felt a slick, warm, melon-size mass: the top of the baby's head. The ensuing thirty seconds of my life have completely disappeared from my mind—I'm not sure I remembered to breathe.

The first thing I recall was a sudden gush of fluid, which I realized was the reason for my spacesuit. I stood there, scared shitless, as I attempted to keep the squirming newborn cradled safely in my arms. People always joked about it being a faux pas for a medical student to drop a baby, but I'd never taken those comments seriously until right then, when I found myself barely able to hold on to the slippery little thing.

"Waaaah!"

Apparently, the infant had inherited his mother's lungs.

The resident took the baby from my hands and placed him on his mother's chest. The mother lay quietly weeping. Still somewhat shell-shocked from what had happened, I had a difficult time concentrating on the resident's directions as I delivered the placenta. Instead, I remained focused on the incredible new life at the head of the bed.

Several minutes later, once we had delivered the placenta and stitched up the small tear in the mother's birth canal, we left the room as quickly as we had entered. I hadn't expected the entire process of birth to move so rapidly. My own mother still teased that after twenty-six years of life I had yet to pay her back for the awful twenty hours she spent in labor. I found her complaint unwarranted, having just participated in my first delivery, which lasted a grand total of thirty seconds.

The resident who had helped me deliver the baby must have recognized my look of shock and amazement, all wrapped up into one wide-eyed expression.

"You did a good job, Jamie," she said. "It's Jamie, right?"

"Uh-huh."

"That was the perfect teaching case. It was her fourth pregnancy and usually, by that point, the baby comes out quickly and easily."

"Uh-huh," I said, still overwhelmed by it all.

"Don't worry. There's no way you could've messed it up, if that's what you're thinking. All you have to do is stand there and catch it. And you'll have plenty more opportunities in the next few days," she said as she turned on her heals and took off toward the next screaming patient's room.

She was right. I caught three more babies that afternoon. They all came into the world as quickly as the first one. With each subsequent delivery, I found myself more aware of what happened during the birthing process. I failed to realize, however, that the babies I delivered were *supposed* to enter the world easily—the resident only let me deliver babies being born by women who had given birth to other children.

The more I thought about how effortless it had been to deliver the four babies without any prior training, the more I realized that, on some level, it made perfect sense. The most basic human process required no instructions—it just happened. Granted, as I would soon learn, not every delivery went so smoothly or so quickly, and many deliveries did require extensive experience on the part of the obstetrician. Nevertheless, I was still amazed that it could happen so easily and so simply.

Later that night, my own mother, a labor and delivery nurse herself, called to wish me a happy twenty-sixth birthday.

"Some way to celebrate your birthday," she said, after I had finished telling her about my eventful day.

Remembering how she always jokingly held it over my head about how much trouble I gave her during labor, I asked, "So, Mom, do you think that twenty-six years is long enough to forgive me for all the pain I caused you?"

"Not a chance," she replied. "Wait until you see the delivery of a firstborn. Then you'll understand why."

"Maybe next year?" I said.

"Yeah, right," she replied.

CHAPTER TWELVE

HELLO, GOOD-BYE

"**P**ULL UP A CHAIR and sit down. The story takes a while to tell," said my new patient, Emily Sokol, in response to my inquiry about the course of her pregnancy. "A few months after I became pregnant with Trevor, our doctor called to tell me that one of the markers in my triple screen had come back abnormal—abnormal, but still nothing to worry myself over until they did some more testing. Once they had looked at Trevor's chromosomes, they arranged to meet with us again, and that's when we found out that he had trisomy eighteen. So a few days later, I went into the office for a sonogram. That's when they discovered that Trevor also had something called myelomeningocele."

She informed me that trisomy eighteen is a severe, life-limiting condition that involves the duplication of a chromosome (for a total of three copies) and results in a whole host of downstream problems, ranging from cardiac defects to breathing problems to, in this case, spinal defects. I vaguely remembered having read about myelomeningocele, in which the skin and bone that normally cover the spinal cord fail to develop. Even though I couldn't remember all the details of trisomy eighteen and myelomeningocele, I did know the bottom-line: none of this was good. Emily confirmed my intuition.

"The doctors told us it was pretty serious. Recently, they've been able to treat it in new ways. That's how I ended up here," she said. "My doctor arranged for me to see a surgeon who performs in utero surgery. The surgeon thought Trevor was a good candidate for the operation. He already did the first part of the procedure."

Her eyes widened, and I think mine did, too. I'd first learned about the relatively new field of fetal surgery while watching a *CNN* special. But I never imagined I might actually meet someone who'd experienced it firsthand, and I definitely never thought I might be present during the delivery of such a baby.

"The surgeon said he was more or less able to repair the hole in the spinal cord. But he is still worried that Trevor might have breathing problems once he comes out. That's why the high-risk obstetricians follow me. They met with Trevor's surgeon and decided to schedule a Cesarean section. They all want to be prepared to take care of Trevor as soon as he enters the world."

I nodded, trying to take this all in.

"And today is the day," she said, her lips quivering ever so slightly as she, probably for the thousandth time that day, realized the enormity of those words.

—-—

Not wanting to miss the opportunity to scrub in on Emily's Cesarean section, I headed back toward the residents' lounge to find the rest of the team. Oddly, no one was in the room. As I stepped back into the hallway, one of the nurses alerted me that everyone was with a fifteen-year-old woman—no, child—who was actively delivering her second baby. In preparation for the possible deliveries that day, I had already read the woman's medical record. I had been amazed to see her young age scribbled across her hospital intake form. I also read that the father was only a mere two years her senior.

By the time I arrived, suited up, and squeezed behind the small crowd of doctors and nurses positioned at the foot of the pregnant woman's bed, I knew it wouldn't be long. By rule of thumb, this one would come quickly and easily.

About thirty seconds later, after the screaming child had rocketed into the world, the father—shoved by his own mother into the space next to the head of the bed—bent over to whisper something in the now not-so-pregnant woman's ear. I imagined his words contained some kind of soothing pleasantry, but instead she looked at him quizzically as if she hadn't understood what he said. He repeated his words a bit more loudly, and this time everyone in the room took note of the exchange.

"I'm hungry. I'm goin' to get some McDonald's. I'll be back later."

Without once looking at his new son, he walked out of the room to the hallway, where a rowdy pack of his friends was waiting. They disappeared noisily down the corridor.

I felt sad for the new mother who had to deal with the experience on her own. But I was more surprised when the mother displayed an equally striking disregard for her new baby. After the resident who delivered the baby finished toweling him off and proudly declared him a healthy baby boy, she went to set the tiny bundle on his mother's chest. Before the resident made it near the side of the bed, however, the mother held up her hand and made a shooing motion with her fingers.

"Do you want to hold him?" the resident asked the mother.

"Nope," the mother replied, turning her attention back to the television hanging in the corner of the hospital room.

Meanwhile, I stood at the side of the newborn's incubator, more interested in the tiny baby. While working in the labor and delivery unit, I usually was stuck with the unglamorous job of delivering the mother's placenta, and I felt increasingly jealous of the pediatricians who examined the newborn. Hovering beside the infant's bassinet, I felt guilty for displaying more excitement to meet the small child than his own mother had. Even more disturbing, I wondered why the mother demonstrated an uncaring attitude. Was she a victim of rape? Did she suffer from severe postpartum depression? Was the true father's identity still under question?

Twenty minutes later, after the fetal surgeon arrived from the children's hospital next door, six of us—the attending obstetrician, the fetal surgeon, the anesthesiologist, two residents, and I—flanked Emily as she lay on the operating table. Her husband wanted to be present for his son's birth, and he stood nervously next to the anesthesiologist. Emily's husband gingerly stroked her loose hair, and he whispered quiet words of encouragement every so often.

"Knife," commanded the attending obstetrician.

"Incision," he said, following the standard operating room protocol of announcing each step of the operation so it could be recorded in the operative record.

Even though I had seen two dozen Cesarean sections during the preceding weeks, the barbaric, yet strangely elegant procedure still amazed me. With one fluid motion, the obstetrician's hand swept across Emily's swollen belly, and the knife left a surprisingly faint red line in its wake. With one more swipe of the knife, the obstetrician sliced through the subcutaneous fat and exposed her abdominal muscles below.

Carefully, the obstetrician separated the layers of muscle, sparing some and slicing through others with the Bovie—an electric knife that burned its way through flesh. The Bovie created a horrible stench. My sole purpose as the medical student in the operating room was to deftly maneuver the suction device to minimize the amount of Bovie smoke making it to the surgeon's nose.

71

Once the obstetrician cut his way through the layers of abdominal tissue, I assumed my only other role—that of holding the retractor. The bladder lay close to the uterus, so the obstetrician needed to prop it carefully out of the way before making a uterine incision. If he wasn't careful, he ran the risk of accidentally nicking the bladder with his knife—and ending up in malpractice court. To spare himself the headache, the surgeon inserted a small metal L-shaped device that pulled the bladder off to the side, and then he connected the handle of the device firmly to the hand of the medical student.

"Hold it right there. And don't move!"

And so it would be recorded in the operative record: "At 0624, the medical student was attached to the retractor device. At 0706, the medical student was removed from the retractor."

Since my job required me to stand behind the obstetrician and reach around him while holding the retractor, all I could see during the remainder of the operation was the green fabric that covered the obstetrician's back.

Some days, when the mood in the operating room was not so tense, the obstetrician and his residents would take advantage of my position and amuse themselves by pimping me with anatomic questions, knowing that I couldn't see anything except their asses.

"What artery is this? How about the name of this ligament?"

I would always stammer the same answer, "Uhhhhhh?"

I was never sure if my constant discomfort in the operating room was because I felt so utterly humiliated, or because the muscles in my back were sore from having held a retractor for the second consecutive hour. Either way, I dreaded standing there.

Today, however, the obstetrician spared me the embarrassment, and he focused on his task of getting Emily's baby into the hands of the awaiting neonatology team.

All of a sudden, I felt a release of pressure on the retractor, which signaled that the baby was either out or nearly out. At this point during every other Cesarean section that I had witnessed, I heard the screaming of a vital newborn. Today, I heard nothing.

"Move, move, move!" the obstetrician ordered. "Come on—get the vacuum on the head! Quickly! Right there. Yes, perfect."

Catching a quick glimpse over the obstetrician's shoulder, I saw him pull a small, blue baby from Emily's open belly. He grasped Trevor in a green surgical towel and then moved swiftly to the head of the table. Earlier that week, understanding that the baby might not survive the delivery, the obstetrician had promised the parents he would let them spend a few moments with Trevor before whisking him away to the neonatal resuscitation bay.

Time stopped. I realized what the obstetrician was doing. It required all my strength to continue holding the bladder retractor. The obstetrician gently rested Trevor on his mother's chest. Almost in unison, Emily and her husband kissed Trevor's tiny head, and Emily said, "Hello, sweet love of mine." The small family locked in an embrace, and they appeared unwilling to let go.

Then, at the polite yet insistent request of the obstetrician, the parents had to say good-bye. The obstetrician picked Trevor up, shuttled him across the room, and took him through the swinging double doors—Trevor was now in the hands of the neonatologists. Still only halfway done with Emily's operation, the obstetrician reentered the operating room, re-gowned and re-gloved, and set to the task of stitching Emily back up.

We worked somberly and quietly throughout the remainder of the operation. Although unspoken, everyone focused on what was happening out beyond the double doors. We all waited for someone to update us about Trevor's status. A nurse stuck her head in through the door, and we all temporarily stopped whatever we were doing.

"We've got the breathing tube in," the nurse said. "His heart is beating strong. We're transferring him to the neonatal intensive care unit now."

Each subsequent time the nurse provided an update, I would glance up from cutting the long ends of sutures to see how Emily and her husband responded to the bit of news. Emily's husband would lean down, kiss her forehead, and lightly whisper, "I love you, honey."

Even from my cramped position, I could see Emily's eyes swell with tears.

Every day during her recovery period, Emily's husband would religiously wheel Emily over to the neonatal intensive care unit to see Trevor. Her spirits were noticeably lifted each time she returned from a visit. By the time Emily was ready to be discharged from the hospital, Trevor had survived his first several days of life. The neonatologists were careful, however, to caution Emily and her husband that Trevor had a difficult and unpredictable course ahead of him. Still, I could see there was unyielding parental hope flickering somewhere behind their eyes.

Soon after I said good-bye to Emily and her husband, our team received an update about the baby born to the teenage parents. A social worker informed us that a childless couple had welcomed the baby into their home. Somewhere deep down inside me, I had expected to hear this. The mother's distant attitude toward the infant and the father's flippant behavior now made perfect sense in this new context. They never intended to keep the baby, and I understood that the outcome demonstrated a different, yet equally devoted kind of love. The teenage parents were more mature than I had initially believed—that's how I decided to think about it for it to make sense.

CHAPTER THIRTEEN

WALK ON BY

ALTHOUGH I DIDN'T REALIZE IT at the time, the several weeks that I had spent on the overnight labor and delivery team had slowly drained my reserve of energy. Looking at myself in the mirror one morning, I noticed that the exhaustion had declared itself again in big black-and-blue bags under my eyes.

Fortunately, I was scheduled to spend a week in the outpatient gynecology clinic before finishing my final two weeks of the rotation in the operating room. I thought back to how rested I felt during my outpatient medicine rotation, and I welcomed the idea of nine-to-five clinic days. I fully intended to store up enough sleep to carry me through those final two weeks of surgery. I'd heard from my classmates that the upcoming gynecologic-oncology surgery rotation was one of the most demanding experiences of third year.

My first morning in the clinic, I arrived at a leisurely 9:00 AM. I expected to see a patient or two per hour, take a generous break for lunch, and then escape early enough to take a jog while it was still light outside. When I found myself staring at a full waiting room—a bursting-at-the-seams kind of full—I knew that I had set myself up for something that would never occur.

In the back of the clinic, I found a frazzled resident running from patient room to patient room. She recognized my short white coat and, obviously overwhelmed by the volume of patients, she hurriedly pulled me aside to offer me a deal.

"Listen. I've seen five patients this morning, and we have another fifteen to see before lunch. It would be really helpful—and a good learning experience—if you could do the histories and physicals for the new patients," she said as if I might have some say in the matter. "Come find me after you're done talking with the first one, and then we'll go back and do the speculum exam together."

Before I could respond, the resident disappeared down the hallway and into another patient's room. I picked up the first chart and leafed through the patient information sheet. My patient was a forty-year-old woman who had no significant past medical history, aside from a bit of occasional heartburn. I figured she was here for her annual OB-GYN visit. It seemed straightforward enough.

I knocked on the patient's door.

"Yes?"

I pushed the door open and peeked in. Having learned my lesson in Dr. Freedman's office, I made sure that the patient was indeed the patient whose chart I held in my hand. An unneeded, incidental knee exam was one thing. In a gynecology clinic, a similar mistake would be unforgivable.

"Ms. Jackson?"

"Yes, that's me."

I edged the rest of my body into the room, held out my hand, and sat down on the small doctor's stool.

"Hi," I said, shaking her hand. "I'm Jamie. I'm a third year medical student. Would you mind if I ask you a few questions about your medical history before the doctor sees you? Is that all right with you?"

"Sure, honey."

"So what brings you into the office today?" I said, falling back on that comfortable, classic doctor question.

"I got a card in the mail telling me to schedule an appointment."

Hmmm. I had the immediate feeling that this was going to be painfully similar to having teeth pulled.

"Do you know what for?"

"Nope."

"This is your first visit to this clinic, right? You've never been here before?"

"Never been here before."

"Did someone refer you here? Maybe your regular doctor?"

"Mmmm. I dunno?"

I was getting nowhere fast, so I decided to try an alternate tactic. Instead of relying on Ms. Jackson to direct the course of the conversation, I figured I would ask her about every gynecologic symptom under the sun. That way, I would almost certainly uncover why her primary medical doctor had sent her to the clinic.

"Have you had any pain, bleeding, spotting, irregular periods, difficulty urinating, burning on urination, itching, or abnormal discharge?" I uttered in one breath.

"Nope," she replied, looking down at her shoes. I was not the only one uncomfortable with the subject matter.

It was the first real sexual health history I had ever taken, aside from the fifteen minutes of practice I'd had during the first year of medical school with a standardized patient—a person who *volunteered* to allow medical students to take her sexual history and then perform an actual speculum exam on her. Although I now felt much more comfortable taking medical histories having spent several months working in the hospital, I still didn't have much experience when it came to asking questions about sex. "Do you have any concerns about your sexual life?" That was about the closest I'd ever come to inquiring about the sensitive subject of sex. Even on the labor and delivery floor, I mostly performed only cursory prenatal sexual histories—I mean, I already knew the answer to the question, "Are you sexually active?"

When it came to obtaining a sexual history, I followed the same advice that I had been given about drawing blood: the quicker the better. I believed this statement based in part on my own trepidation and in part on how uncomfortable I assumed the questions would make the woman.

"How about your pregnancies? You have two children? Have you been pregnant more than twice? Were they normal, vaginal births? Any complications?"

"I've got two children."

"Are you sexually active?"

"Nope."

"Do you use any birth control or protection when you are?" I said, my voice shaking.

"I just told you I ain't."

"Any history of sexually transmitted diseases?" I bit my tongue. They had taught us to use the phrase "sexually transmitted infections." It did sound slightly less threatening, but it was too late.

"No," she said, growing visibly annoyed.

"Are you concerned that you might have any infections right now?"

"No! Don't you listen, child?"

Flustered, I apologized, and then I thrust a patient gown toward her.

"Could you put this on? I'll be back shortly with the doctor."

"Mm-hmm."

I rose from my seat and bolted for the door—the encounter had gone exactly as I thought it would. I felt more uncomfortable knowing that I would have to come back and perform a gynecologic exam on Ms. Jackson.

As I waited for the resident outside of Ms. Jackson's room, I scribbled the results of my brief interrogation on a blank page in Ms. Jackson's chart. After a few minutes, the resident emerged from another room and headed my way.

"So, what's she got?"

"Nothing, actually. She's not sexually active, she's not pregnant, and she denied the entire gynecologic review of symptoms," I responded. "I think she's just here for an annual check-up."

"Nothing? No one's ever here for nothing," she said curtly. "Follow me."

We reentered Ms. Jackson's room in a grand bustle. I kept my eyes directed toward the ground. The resident introduced herself and then, as she prepared the exam tray, decided to ask several quick questions herself.

"Are you sexually active, Ms. Jackson?"

Having already told the resident that Ms. Jackson wasn't sexually active, I was slightly offended by her repetition of the question, especially after the trouble I'd encountered.

"Yes."

I looked up from the floor and stared directly at Ms. Jackson's face in disbelief. She gazed ahead and smiled sweetly at the resident.

"How many partners?"

"Well, that's why I'm here. Just two, but I think one of 'em has been cheatin' on me," Ms. Jackson continued. "I got this itch starting last week. Down there."

"Okay, I'll see what we can do," replied the resident. "I'm going to examine you and take some swabs to see if you've got an infection."

The resident shot me an "I told you so" look, and I wished that I might spontaneously combust right there and then. My face seemed to be burning hot enough to ignite a fire.

I had just experienced, firsthand, the touted curse of the medical student: a patient matter-of-factly tells a medical student one thing and then, once a *real* doctor has entered the room, she reveals her full story. Other medical students had warned me that this might happen, but that afternoon I discovered for myself that the curse was a true phenomenon, and in this case, it was exaggerated by the sensitive nature of the subject matter.

For the remainder of the week, I attempted to hone my history-taking skills. I tried out different approaches, styles, and permutations of questions to see if I could elicit the same answers that the real doctor would eventually get. No matter how hard I tried to unravel a patient's story before the attending physician came in the room, my attempts were uniformly unsuccessful, and it left me feeling angry at those patients who actively resisted including me in the process.

On the last day of my duty in the clinic, I was surprised when a patient complained right from the start about her irregular menstrual bleeding. I had just read the list of different possible diagnoses for this symptom, so I felt especially prepared to interview the woman. Maybe I might come up with my own diagnosis.

"When did this begin?"

"A few days ago."

"Are you pregnant?"

"No."

"Any history of bleeding in the past? Irregular periods?"

"No."

"Are you taking any medications or hormones?"

"No."

We went back and forth like this for a few minutes. Certain that the curse had once again set in, I resorted to seeing if maybe she could diagnose the problem herself.

"Do you have any idea why this might be happening?"

"Well, I took some of those pills. The ones you take when you don't want to be pregnant anymore."

Okay, now we were getting somewhere—although I was uncertain how to handle this new information.

"I started bleeding yesterday, and it hasn't stopped yet," she said. "And now I'm having quite a bit of pain."

Knowing I was out of my league, I cut the interview short, excused myself, and hurried outside to track down my resident. We returned to the room to examine the woman.

With the woman reclined on the exam table and her legs situated in the stirrups, the resident set to work and began a speculum exam. As she did, blood ran down the woman's leg, snaked down the side of the table, and then pooled on the linoleum flooring at the foot of the table. The bright red-on-white looked almost like a Japanese flag.

My eyes concentrated on the resident's hands, which seemed to be pulling something from the woman. A few moments later, I realized that a lump of flesh, stringy and soft, lay in the center of the pool of blood. The discolored tissue did not have the vitality of the surrounding bright red blood. It just lay there on the white floor, an unglamorous resting place.

"Here, switch places with me," said the resident.

I hesitated.

"Come on, hurry up."

We shuffled positions, and she placed the pair of forceps firmly against my gloved hands.

"There, can you see that?" she asked. "Yes, that's right. Grab it with the forceps, but don't pull on it with too much pressure. If it doesn't come out easily, don't force it."

The patient squirmed. Her fingers gripped the sides of the table, and the weight of her body crunched the white tissue paper beneath her, which was the loudest sound in the otherwise silent room. Covered in sweat and blood, the paper drape faintly reminded me of a finger-painting project.

My hands shook. I could barely focus on my simple task. I sat with my gaze focused on the drops of blood pooling on the floor beneath me. I was unable to look straight ahead.

My hesitation betrayed promises I had previously made to myself: I would provide the care that my patients needed, period. My own beliefs were supposed to stop at the door. That's what

I had told myself. Yet, I sat there paralyzed thinking about the service I was asked to provide.

Clearly in pain, the woman continued to writhe on the table. Swallowing the bile rising in my throat, I looked. The other half of the lump of tissue sat between the bills of the speculum. Following the resident's instructions, I numbly maneuvered the forceps, grasped the puddle of bloody flesh between the steel jaws, and pulled out the remaining tissue.

"Good, we're all done here," said the resident, trying to reassure both the patient and me. "You might have some bleeding and pain for the next few days, but we got the majority of it out. If you have fever or any heavy bleeding, you should come back to the clinic. Any questions?"

"Nope."

The tone of the exchange surprised me—it felt exceedingly inadequate for what had just taken place. It seemed like the kind of dialogue that might occur between a mechanic and a car owner. I think we all would have benefited from a group counseling session, although none of us wanted to utter a word.

Several minutes later, the woman walked out of the room. She was fully clothed, no longer open and fragile beneath her too-small hospital gown. She was a woman on her way to work, a woman you might pass on the street without giving her a second thought.

"Bye," she mumbled to me.

"Bye," I said as she walked out.

Afterward, I locked myself in the men's bathroom. I needed the quiet. While I sat there thinking, I realized that people would pass me by, too, without seeing me—I mean, really seeing me. No one would know what I had just done, or that I was trembling beneath my skin.

All three of us in that examining room had hidden behind our words and our actions. In the same way that so many other patients had done that week, I would have gladly told a lie had anyone asked me how I was doing. "I'm great. Really," I would have answered, when inside I was shaken up and scared, trying to figure out what I had just done. Maybe by maintaining that facade I was attempting to convince myself that I would be okay. Maybe that's exactly how I would make good on my promise.

Chapter Fourteen

Lift

ONE WEEK LATER, at the shockingly early morning hour of 5:00 AM, I had my first real encounter with him. He stood there, his long white coat starched and gleaming white—almost enough to blind me in the early morning darkness of the hospital corridors. I had just begun the grueling surgical conclusion to my obstetrics rotation.

"I only want him to operate on me. He's the best. I mean look at him—he's perfect," a patient had insisted the previous evening. I had to admit, Dr. Greenwald's immaculate appearance did give the impression that nothing *ever* went wrong in his presence. From the clean lines of his coat to his expertly honed physique, he exuded perfection.

Still, I'd heard grumblings from my fellow students: "He doesn't talk to anyone lower in rank than a supervising resident. Don't expect to be acknowledged." In my mind, I had formed an image of a tyrant who ruled his minions with a wicked hand. At least he appeared to be a respectable-looking tyrant.

Trying to remain calm in his imposing presence, I focused on the laboratory values that I had jotted down on a sheet of paper just minutes earlier. Although my mind felt as if it were still asleep, I was able to muster enough energy to recite properly the strings of numbers for the group. (Surgical rounds required little thought on the part of the medical student, which was fortunate, since 5:00 AM was far too early for most people to make sense of anything.)

While I spewed the laboratory results for a patient named Emma Spedding, I realized that there had been truth in the warnings from my classmates. Even though my presentation of the patient lab values placed me on center stage, only three of the four available pairs of eyes acknowledged my presence. The fourth pair of eyes—Dr. Greenwald's—wandered aimlessly, pausing momentarily on just about everything else in the hallway except my figure, clad in my short white coat. When I finished recounting the laboratory values, I was surprised to hear the voice of Dr. Greenwald—he had broken his strict rule of not speaking to medical students.

"She has metastatic, stage four cancer. I saw her CT yesterday. She's going to die. Period. So tell me, why do we spend so much time each morning outside this room? Let's get on with it already."

Was I supposed to answer that question? Then, I realized he was addressing the resident standing next to me. And the question was rhetorical, which spared her the shame of having to acknowledge his cold, unfeeling statement. Despite feeling thankful that no one, including me, had to answer his question, I feared that since we were standing directly outside the patient's door, she might have overheard her doctor's comment. My emotions sprang to life. I imagined how appalled I would feel hearing my own fate described in cold, sterile language.

"Let's go! We have a case at seven AM," Dr. Greenwald said. With that, he spun on his heels and started toward the next patient's room at a brisk pace.

The group scurried down the hallway to catch up with Dr. Greenwald's billowing white coattails. While he stood outside the doorway of the next patient and repeated the process all over again, I bit at my lower lip trying to determine if I should say something. I thought, "Surely this kind of remark cannot be condoned. But how can I possibly make any difference as a lowly medical student?" I searched the faces of the other members of the team, and I tried to assess if anyone else shared my shock at the attending physician's callous comments. No one else looked surprised. I assumed that most of the team had worked with Dr. Greenwald on prior occasions and knew better than to say anything. Whether they remained silent because they felt that having a cohesive team was most important for providing good patient care, or because they were scared to raise their concerns (as I was), I understood the message: "Fall into line, keep your mouth shut, and we'll all be better off."

The supervising resident, unlike his boss, acknowledged my presence and sensed my concern. He caught my gaze and gave me a stern look. With his eyes, he silently said, "Calm down. We'll talk about this later." I took his unspoken advice, pushed the incident to the back of my mind, and numbly continued to read numbers from my list of laboratory values, all the while wishing for the morning to end.

The week wore on in a similar vein. Each morning, we would begin rounds at an ungodly hour, followed by a full day's worth of surgery, and end with more rounds in the evening. To survive the brutally long days, I'd learned that it was often easier to accept Dr. Greenwald's inappropriate actions and comments. I found myself constantly wishing that this rotation would end. Everything about it was miserable.

It didn't help my down-in-the-dumps mood that the patients whom we cared for had terrible prognoses and often equally awful qualities of life. Many of the women had spent much of their recent existences in the hospital hooked up to intravenous lines too numerous to count, while lying in bed, withered, nauseated, and exhausted. As much as I resisted acknowledging

Dr. Greenwald's matter-of-fact way of thinking, I knew that many, if not all, of the women *would* eventually die—probably sooner than later. I'd discovered that by the time a patient made it to Dr. Greenwald's waiting room, she had often exhausted every other treatment option with her previous oncologists.

Toward the end of the first week, I learned that Dr. Greenwald had scheduled a twenty-two-year-old patient for the removal of a teratoma—a strange, but harmless ovarian tumor that contains many types of human tissue, including teeth, bones, and skin. I found myself drawn to witness her surgery, but not for the obvious reason. It was, perhaps, the only surgery I would experience during my two weeks of gynecologic-oncology surgery where the patient would be expected to recover fully without any long-term effects.

In the operating room, everyone was hopeful and good-spirited. We readied the young woman for her surgery. After the anesthesiologist had put the patient to sleep, Dr. Greenwald swooshed into the room and assumed his normal position at the side of the operating table. While he waited for the scrub nurse to tie his gown closed, he took the opportunity to greet the anesthesiologist, the residents, and the rest of the operating room staff—he did not look my way once.

Even though I childishly wanted to boycott Dr. Greenwald by ignoring his presence, I was too interested in watching a curative surgery. His hands worked quickly. Within a few minutes, Dr. Greenwald exposed the grapefruit-size mass hanging off the patient's right ovary. Expertly, he sliced open the small capsule containing the tumor, plucked it out, and tossed it into a specimen bag beside the table. I watched in awe. In terms of performing the surgery, he was every bit as amazing as people had said. I wondered if I had judged him too harshly.

Then he realized the tumor had damaged too much of the patient's right ovary for it to remain viable. Dr. Greenwald swore under his breath and decided he would have to take out the ovary. With a few more deft swipes of his hand, the patient's ovary was tossed into the specimen bag alongside the tumor. Then he broke the silence.

"It's not like she'll need this anyway."

We all looked up from under our masks and wondered what in the world he meant.

"She's a lesbian," he clarified, laughing. "So she won't need it."

Silence.

Seething, raging, boiling silence.

———

By the end of my second week, I was tired and angry. I hated standing in the operating room, which made up a large portion of how I spent my day. Even worse, I hated being in the operating room with Dr. Greenwald. To that end, I avoided the operating room at all costs, and I devised a plan to keep out of there by volunteering to do "scut work" on the floors. Scut work entailed running samples of blood to the lab or recording the outputs of patients' tubes and catheters. For the most part, the plan worked. Although I still spent the same total number of hours per day in the hospital, on the days that I visited with patients instead of standing idly in the operating room, I found that the time passed faster. And, what's more, I felt satisfied at the end of the day.

One afternoon, I went to check on the patient whom Dr. Greenwald had labeled a "goner" my first day. After I knocked on Emma Spedding's door, I introduced myself.

"Come in, please," she said in a fragile voice.

As I entered, I noticed a small, plastic toy soldier coiled in Emma's fingers. She held it to her chest in the same telling way that a frightened child clutches her worn teddy bear, as if it might offer some protection against the darkness of night.

"Hi, Ms. Spedding. I was wondering if it would be all right if I did a brief physical exam."

"I'm kind of tired and a touch down, honey. I don't know. Maybe later?" she replied glumly. I could see she was worn out from a long day of tests to evaluate the effects of her chemotherapy.

Exhausted myself, I didn't insist. Instead, I offered my assistance in untangling the thicket of strings that attached a small, plastic parachute to the toy soldier's back. She accepted my help.

After a bit of questioning, I discovered that her youngest grandchild had left the toy behind while visiting her that morning. Although she knew he'd miss it, she seemed deeply relieved by its presence. In her drab, muted-green hospital room, the small toy provided a reminder of her grandson's bright smile—it would help combat the quiet emptiness of nighttime in the hospital.

In a soft voice, she continued to describe her grandson while I worked. Then, holding the newly extricated soldier to her chest, she confided in me.

"I've always wanted to parachute."

"Me too," I replied.

After that simple exchange, I sensed an immediate shift in her mood.

"Why don't you come back to my room later once things have quieted down," she said with a different energy in her voice. "I could use your help with something. And make sure to bring my wheelchair—I want to get out of this gloomy room for a little while."

She spoke with the grin of a mischievous child—the same kind of look that I used to give my mother while vehemently denying that I had raided the candy jar, never mind the streaks of sweet chocolate around the corners of my mouth.

Several hours later, bleary-eyed but still intrigued by Emma's mysterious request, I returned to her room with a wheelchair in tow. Despite my quizzical looks and repeated inquiries, she remained tight-lipped and refused to tell me where we were going or what we were doing.

"Can I at least tell the nurse where we'll be?" I said, pleading with Emma.

"Shush."

With an outstretched finger, she eagerly directed me down corridor after corridor until we reached the three-story atrium overlooking the hospital's main lobby.

"There. Stop!"

I surveyed our surroundings. She had positioned us next to the glass railing of the atrium's balcony.

"Look," Emma said as she relaxed her clenched fist and produced the tiny toy soldier. Her excited hands fumbled to unwind the strings that attached the small, plastic parachute to the soldier's body, and then she looked up at me with her gleaming eyes.

Anticipating her plan, innocent as it was, I glanced nervously at the security guard seated below us at the visitor's desk.

"Don't worry, honey—I'll take all the blame. You just do as I say."

With that, the small, elderly woman took one final look around to make sure no witnesses were present. Then, with a quick swipe of her frail, bony hand, she sent the toy soldier careening over the glass railing and out into the empty space beyond.

The soldier's camouflaged parachute unfolded, billowing above him, and safely carried him down through three stories of air to the ground below. Emma could no longer contain her excitement. She giggled in the infectious, full-bellied way that children do—that giddy kind of laughter that cannot be contained. I started laughing, too.

Once we each caught our breath, she urgently instructed, "Go, go—GO!" And we took off like Bonnie and Clyde, the white-coated medical student and his elderly, wheelchair-bound patient, laughing hysterically as we raced down the hall and away from the scene of the crime. We might have gotten away scot-free had we remembered to recover the crucial piece of evidence that we had left behind.

Later that night, on my way out of the hospital, I tried to slink past the security guard sitting in the main lobby, but his voice stopped me.

"This yours?" he said with a sly smile.

Embarrassed, I grabbed the small figure and made a beeline for the door. Once I was outside, I started to laugh again.

After rounds ended the next morning, I walked into Emma's sunshine-filled room along with her nurse.

"How are you this morning?" I said, noticing a brilliant new glow in Emma's face.

"Just lovely, dear," she responded, and her eyes twinkled. "I dreamed I was flying last night."

After we finished, I slid the small, plastic soldier onto Emma's bedside table. An impish grin spread across her face. From the doorway, I could hear Emma's nurse playfully inquiring about what trouble we had gotten ourselves into, and Emma giggling as she replied, "I plead the Fifth!"

"Me too," I called from the hallway. I smiled to myself and wondered what new adventure she would dream up next. I promised myself that for the remainder of my rotation, I would try to keep my spirits high—if not for myself, then for the sake of patients like Emma.

Emma provided me with the golden answer to the question I asked myself after spending my first day with Dr. Greenwald: "How can I possibly make any difference as a lowly medical student?" Although I still didn't feel comfortable to so much as utter a word in Dr. Greenwald's presence, I now realized that a hundred of his stinging comments could not survive for long in the presence of a single, smiling face.

PEDIATRICS

Chapter Fifteen

Eyes Wide Open

"**N**O, DON'T MAKE ME GO out there! Nooooo!"
I imagined this might be the last thought going through a baby's mind before he entered this world. I had seen a few dozen deliveries during the past two months, and the babies' angry wails seemed to lend weight to my theory. Whenever a labor lasted an especially long time, I joked that the problem didn't result from the mother's anatomy (the most common cause of prolonged labor), but instead was a result of a baby digging in his heels and hanging on for dear life, not wanting to leave his warm, nurturing home.

Much in the same way, I dreaded my transitions from service to service and from rotation to rotation, which occurred every few weeks. Just when I had begun to feel settled with one routine, I would have to abandon my comfortable world and face the harsh unfamiliarity of another. Granted, the past two weeks on the gynecologic-oncology surgery service had left me ready to move on to something new. Still, there was always that initial transition period that required a good deal of effort to navigate—without any guarantee that the time and energy would be worthwhile. Each time I faced the idea of having to join a new team, I found myself mimicking the babies whom I had helped deliver. "Hell no, don't make me go! Nooooo!"

Truthfully, nothing bad ever happened during these transitions—at least, nothing to warrant such dread on my part. If anything, the first few days of a new rotation were the easiest days. No one ever expected much from me or gave me much responsibility. My only real task consisted of figuring out the nuances and preferences of the new team. Still, however innocuous those initial few days should have been, I consistently found these transitional experiences uncomfortable to navigate.

By the time I reported to meet my new team on the inpatient general pediatrics ward, I had developed an awful feeling in the pit of my stomach. I expected to find a group of shiny, happy people (the common stereotype of pediatricians). But this group seemed to be at least as bleary-eyed and tired, if not more so, than the obstetrics residents with whom I had just finished working. The previous night, like most spring nights at a major pediatric hospital, had been a busy one with dozens of children suffering from coughs, colds, and the flu.

Judging by everyone's confused looks during the beginning of rounds, I realized that the rest of the team—the interns, the residents, and the attending physician—had also just started a new rotation. It made for absolute chaos that morning. No one knew the patients, and no one knew one another. Some treaded lightly, afraid to offend any of their new coworkers, and others made their views plainly known, as if to establish their foothold early on. Fortunately, as an ancillary member of the team, I sat unnoticed at the edge of the mess.

By the time team rounds ended, an uneasy feeling had overtaken me, much like the one I had that first day of my internal medicine rotation. I felt overwhelmed by the newness of everything: unfamiliar terminology to learn, endless corridors and hallways to navigate, an unfriendly and foreign computer system, different sounds (shrieking children and irate, scared parents), and an entirely new team. I found myself questioning yet again: "Why on earth did I willingly decide to subject myself to this process of becoming a doctor?" Before I could settle into having my own practice someday, I would have to endure at least four more years of training—and of bouncing from one experience to another.

Later that morning on my way to a lecture, I serendipitously bumped into Dr. Brixton, one of my professors from the first two years of medical school. Dr. Brixton was a pediatrician who had gained role model status in my mind. He smiled and welcomed me to the children's hospital, but then he hesitated as he noticed my less-than-stellar mood.

"Come on. I'm gonna buy you a cup of coffee. Let's go talk."

Although he looked like he had somewhere to be, he put his hand on my back and ushered me down the hallway toward the cafeteria. As we walked, he dialed a number on his cell phone, and then he instructed his own team that he would be late to rounds—something had come up.

"So what's going on?" he said, turning his attention back to me.

"Not much, other than I hate being a medical student right now," I responded. "I feel like every time I start to get the hang of things—just when I can start to make tiny differences in patients' lives—the rotation ends, and I am back at square one. Game over, try again."

He nodded.

"Sometimes I think I'll never feel settled until I'm an attending physician with my own practice," I said. "And that's a really, really long time away—not to make you feel old or anything. I'm just not sure that I'm going to be able to survive medicine for that long."

"I've got news for you," he said. "Being an attending physician doesn't make it any easier. Sure, I have a bit more experience under my belt, and I don't have to worry like you do about making giant leaps between the different fields of medicine, but I still have to deal with the same old shit. I encounter a new combination of residents, medical students, and nurses every time I am on service. And believe me, it doesn't get any more difficult than being the one in charge of making sure that the team runs smoothly. With ten years of experience under my belt, those first few days are always chaotic and often a bit terrifying."

"Any tips?" I asked.

"Yeah. I've learned to chalk it up to the 'Oh, shit' factor," he said.

"Huh?"

"Listen, that feeling—the uncomfortable, chaotic one—I still get it every time I start working with a new team or step into a room of an especially complicated patient. That's the 'Oh, shit' factor. But, I've come to expect it and I've learned that—and this is the real beauty of it—the feeling usually disappears after a couple of days. Most of the time, I end up wondering what I was scared of in the first place. The times that the feeling doesn't disappear— that's when I know there's something I need to work on."

I began to see what he was getting at.

"That's the power of the 'Oh, shit' factor," he continued. "You know it's going to happen, but you also know it will pass. This way, I make sure to cut myself a little slack those first few days of something new, and I know that, most times, things will improve."

The simple brilliance of his idea made perfect sense to me. When I reflected on the preceding several months, I realized that the first few days of each new rotation had indeed been the most difficult: on the internal medicine ward, at Dr. Freedman's office, on the labor and delivery ward, and in the operating room. The unmistakable pattern seemed impossible to have missed. Dr. Brixton's "Oh, shit" theory explained it perfectly.

"I buy it," I said. "I'll ride it out for a few more days before I go making any rash decisions."

He smiled as he stood up from the table.

"If you still feel unsettled with things by the end of the week, we can talk again," he said. "But for now—damn, man—chill out, and give yourself a break. Have a little confidence that things will work out. You're going to be just fine. Okay?"

"Sure."

"And if I don't get to rounds soon, I think I'm going to make a lot of people on my new team anxious. I've got to go," he said, and he took off down the hallway.

———

I called my mom later that night and recounted the wisdom that Dr. Brixton had shared with me. The funny thing is, it was the same advice my mother had been giving me all along during our phone conversations, just packaged with different words. Only later, after I had talked with her, would I realize how gracious she'd been to step aside and let me give Dr. Brixton all the credit.

Before we hung up, she made a suggestion that was part Mom and part labor and delivery nurse.

"Promise me you'll go walk by the newborn nursery sometime tomorrow. Just look at the babies for a little while, and tell me you don't think that they're the most beautiful things in the world. They'll make you smile, regardless of how the rest of your day goes."

The next morning, I followed my mom's advice and took a detour by the newborn unit. As I stood there gazing through the glass nursery window, I had to admit that, although I had firsthand knowledge of how much the babies screamed when they came out, the newborns appeared much happier after a day or two of adjusting to the life of snugly blankets, cooing parents, and all the attention they could stand. Dr. Brixton had probably gotten to them, too! I imagined him cradling the pouting newborns, counseling them as he had done for me, but phrasing it slightly differently. "It'll get better, I promise," I could hear him whisper in their ears. I laughed to myself, deciding that if the tiny newborns could survive one of life's greatest transitions, then I could survive a few more days until I felt steady on my feet again.

Chapter Sixteen

Setting Sights

A LTHOUGH I DID FIND my stride in a few days, I realized that a safe and quick passage through a rough spell was not always the rule—two of the team's new patients had endured particularly tumultuous transitions in their lives. The first, an Amish infant, had arrived at the hospital gravely ill, and according to his local community doctor, had suffered from infection after infection during his first several months of life. The second, another infant, had initially fared better, thriving and growing like a baby should, but he had recently begun to have daily seizures.

As I listened during rounds that morning, I could tell by the tone of the conversation that both of the infants were far sicker than any of the other patients were that I had seen during the previous week. Because neither of the infants carried a definite diagnosis, the management of their symptoms did not follow the straightforward treatments for patients admitted for things like asthma or gastroenteritis. Instead, the attending physician and residents tossed around the foreign-sounding names of diseases and syndromes of which I had either never heard or which I had only seen printed obscurely in the "Suggested Supplementary Readings" sections at the end of textbook chapters.

My new, bleary-eyed supervising resident seized the opportunity to make good use of a new medical student, and he assigned me to canvass the current medical literature for information about each of the suspected diagnoses. Even though I knew the job was not a particularly glamorous one, I enjoyed feeling as if I might contribute something to the care of a patient. At the same time, I also felt slightly anxious. Up until this point, my presentations of information had always been an exercise intended for my own education. Judging by the serious nature of morning rounds, I felt like the patients' health might depend, in part, on how thoroughly I researched the possible diagnoses. Maybe I was fooling myself into feeling more important than I was, but I still approached the task with a newfound determination.

Before sending me in the direction of the library, the supervising resident pulled me aside. He wanted to introduce me to the two, little patients and their families. As soon as I walked into the first infant's room, my novice eyes could tell that Simon, the small nine-month-old Amish patient, was ill.

Never having interacted with an Amish family before, I followed the lead of the more seasoned supervising resident. I shook hands with the father, and I nodded courteously at the mother. Then, I nudged up against Simon's steel-railed hospital bed and introduced myself to the tiny bundle. After a few moments, he turned his weary head to meet my gaze. I could see the sickness behind his eyes—those same "I'm-not-feeling-so-good" eyes my mother had told me that as a parent, she trusted more than a thermometer.

The supervising resident sidled up against the opposite railing of the crib, and we carefully unwrapped little Simon from his cocoon of baby blankets. Talking quietly, so as not to alarm the parents, the resident explained key things I needed to look for when examining an infant. He pointed to Simon's belly and the resident's eyes grew wide as if to say, "Make note of this, but wait until we're in the hallway before we talk about it." Simon's abdomen was as wide as he was long. I felt along the right side of his stomach where the bottom edge of the liver is usually palpable, but all I could feel was his firm, swollen belly.

We finished examining Simon, rewrapped him in his blankets, and exited the room. Out in the hallway, the resident assured me that I might never see such a swollen abdomen again.

"You should go back later. Do a more thorough abdominal exam, and focus on trying to figure out the size of his liver—it's gigantic," he said as we approached the doorway of the next patient. "But for now, see if you can find the next patient's physical abnormality."

When we entered the room, I noticed that Owen, the other nine-month-old infant, had propped himself up in a classic baby position. His arms stretched out beside him like airplane wings, and they formed a tripod with the rest of his body. His wobbly head teetered at a precarious balancing point, and it seemed as if he would either give into the relentless pull of gravity or muster the strength to look upward. He chose the latter, and with a herculean effort, he lifted his head and fixed his eyes on the world in front of him. As if supremely proud of his accomplishment, Owen's chubby face beamed with the widest smile I have ever seen.

Honestly, I don't think I could have imagined a healthier looking baby. Where Simon had instantly appeared sick, Owen exuded the kind of energy and playfulness that I expected from an infant his age. His cheeks glowed with vital, rosy patches of color, and he cooed, smiled, and flirted with his new audience.

I convinced myself that Owen's parents had been overzealous in bringing their son to the hospital. I knew he'd had a few, brief seizures during the preceding days, but after witnessing his playfulness, I honestly didn't think about them as being part of his diagnosis.

After we concluded our visit with Owen, the supervising resident asked if I had noticed the significant physical finding.

Sheepishly, I admitted that I hadn't found anything out of the ordinary.

"Did you notice anything odd about his hair?"

"Nope." Really? His hair?

"The next time you go back in the room, rub his head. See what you feel, okay?"

I replied that I would, although I still wondered what in the world could possibly be wrong with the child's hair. Why had it caused such concern? Instead of studying the infant's chart more thoroughly, as I should have done, I tracked down a dictionary to look up the word "cherub." That morning during rounds, the team had used the term "cherubic facies" when they spoke about Owen. I discovered that he fit the description perfectly: his chubby cheeks and golden locks resembled those of an angel.

Later, while sitting in the library, I read from a section of a textbook devoted to human copper metabolism. The attending physician suspected that Owen suffered from a rare disease that affected how the body processed copper. My eyes skimmed the pages and stopped on the phrase "Menke's Kinky Hair Disease." As I read on, I realized why the attending physician had suspected the disorder in Owen's case: its manifestations included seizures, bone disease, lack of skin and hair pigmentation, and—most notably—brittle, kinky hair.

The disease had no cure, and it was uniformly fatal. After a relatively normal first year of life, an affected patient would experience a rapid degeneration of his neurological system, and this deterioration would culminate in death. Nevertheless, realizing that Menke's kinky hair disease occurred infrequently, I chose to believe in the disorder's innocence until proven guilty—despite how closely Owen's symptoms fit the disorder.

Next, I turned my attention to the suspected cause of little Simon's illness. Unlike Menke's kinky hair disease, I had heard the name of his disorder before—chronic granulomatous disease (CGD). Although also uncommon, I read that this genetic disorder of the white blood cells did occur more frequently among Amish populations. It also happened to fit Simon's symptoms like a glove. CGD results in the inability of white blood cells— the infection fighting cells—to kill bacteria in the body, which predisposes the body to developing overwhelming infections similar to the one in Simon's abdomen. Children who are exposed to higher levels of bacteria face an increased risk for developing severe infections. Being Amish, Simon's family did not process or pasteurize any of their homegrown products, including milk and honey, which Simon ate routinely. Nevertheless, therapy with antibiotics usually allowed affected patients to live relatively normal lives, and the prognosis was still favorable. In severe cases, a bone marrow transplant was curative for the disease.

After I concluded my research and put the final changes on my presentations for the rest of the team, I made a quick stop by Owen's room before I left for home. While I sat and chatted with his parents, Owen smiled gleefully as I played peekaboo with him. When I said good-bye to both Owen and his parents, I reached down to tousle his hair. Indeed, it had the rough texture of steel wool, just as the textbook had described.

While I walked home in the warm spring air, I considered the two infant's suspected diagnoses. If the attending physician's suspicions were correct, the infant who looked so sick would live a relatively healthy life, while the infant who looked so vital would probably not live to see another spring.

—————

The confirmatory tests for each infant's tentative diagnosis took several days to return from the laboratory. In the meantime, the attending physician started Simon on antibiotics, and his general appearance improved tremendously. Owen's parents spent yet another day waiting and wondering, and they prayed that their son would not have another seizure. The attending physician had asked Owen's parents not to search the Internet until the medical team had a chance to gather additional clinical information. He wanted to avoid needless worry on their part in case they started reading about Menke's kinky hair disease and its dismal prognosis, only to have the diagnostic test come back negative. The parents agreed to hold off, but I could only imagine how difficult it must have been for Owen's parents to let their minds run wild with fear while they waited for additional definitive information.

Simon's test results came back first. As expected, he had CGD. That same day, we arranged a meeting time with the family to discuss the new diagnosis. Later, once the family and the medical team had assembled in the small meeting room, it surprised me when the physician—the one who had so carefully pieced the information together—described the new diagnosis in a matter-of-fact manner and without any visible emotion. I knew that he had retired from the military several years earlier, and I imagined that he had probably addressed his soldiers in much the same way as he did his current staff: with firm words, a reserved temperament, and supreme confidence.

Simon's parents nodded, and if anything, they appeared visibly relieved and maybe even joyous. During the previous several days, while talking with family members, Simon's parents had discovered that two of his estranged uncles also suffered from CGD. Both uncles were alive and healthy. I realized that it probably hadn't mattered how bluntly the attending physician had broken the news—Simon's parents had prepared themselves for the diagnosis, and they knew that their son would almost certainly continue to live a relatively normal life.

Owen's test also came back positive. In his case, however, his parents did not have the benefit of hearing surviving family members' favorable testimonials. Still adhering to the doctor's suggestion that they avoid looking for information on the Internet, Owen's parents only knew that their son might have an uncommon genetic disorder. Up to this point, I wasn't sure anyone had raised the concern that Owen might have a fatal condition. I was sure, however, that the thought had crossed their minds while they anxiously awaited more information.

When I heard the results of Owen's test from the supervising resident, I immediately thought, "Who is going to break the news to the family?" Having witnessed the emotionless manner in which the attending physician had communicated Simon's diagnosis, I felt extremely uncomfortable to think about the gruff man delivering the news to Owen's anxious parents. I thought they needed—and deserved—someone who would provide empathy and compassion, not stoic detachment.

As the attending physician walked into Owen's room to give the diagnosis, I braced myself both mentally and physically. At least I would learn how *not* to break bad news. The physician squeezed in next to Owen's parents on a tiny couch in the hospital room. I looked at the attending physician's face and noticed a tear had rolled down his face. I watched the drop pause for a moment at the edge of his chin, and then take a brave plunge into the space below. Even before the tear reached its final resting place on the physician's starched, long white coat, the soft sniffles of the grieving parents and the military-trained physician filled the room.

Twice that week, I had forgotten that all-important rule: "Never judge a book by its cover." I made assumptions that incorrectly guided my initial perceptions about the health of the two infants. I also questioned the compassion and sensitivity of their physician (whom I stereotyped as an incredibly intelligent, but unfeeling man).

On some level, I knew I couldn't have anticipated what lurked deeply within the infants' genetic codes or behind the starched, impassive shell of the attending physician's demeanor. Only with time could I discover the hidden, deeper truths. Nevertheless, I had a choice to make whenever my mind teetered at that precarious balancing point, deciding whether to pass judgment on a situation: I could either succumb to the relentless lure of drawing quick conclusions, or I could lift my head—although it might sometimes require a herculean effort—and smile indiscriminately on the world. As Owen had, I hoped that I would always find the strength to do the latter.

Chapter Seventeen

Too Much Information

SOMETHING VIBRATED AGAINST MY HIP. The sensation jolted me out of the half-sleep I had fallen into during the last hour of rounds. It took me a few additional moments before I realized that my pager had gone off. No one ever paged me. And, if someone had, the only people who knew how to use the paging system were all sitting beside me. As I read the small, flashing characters displayed on the pager's screen, I sucked in a deep breath—it was my mother's cell phone number. I had never given my mother my pager number.

I assumed the worst, and I felt certain that something awful had happened—an illness-or-death kind of awful. The faces of my father and my brother appeared in my mind, and I had a sick feeling that one of them—or worse, both of them—had been injured or killed in an accident. Shaken, I stood and excused myself from the room.

"Sorry, I have to use the bathroom," I whispered as the residents moved their knees and feet out of my way. I settled on this particular excuse, certain that telling the truth about who paged me would elicit laughter and mocking looks. Everyone knew that medical students rarely received important pages—certainly not the kind that warranted interrupting rounds.

After I found a phone at the nurses' station, I dialed my mom's cell phone number. She picked up right away.

"Jamie?"

I could tell by her voice that she'd been crying.

"Grandma just called me," she said. "They found a mass in her lung at the doctor's office today."

I swallowed, selfishly relieved that nothing was wrong with my mother or father or brother, but then I found myself teary-eyed once I realized that my grandma was sick. She was the one person I called every Friday night to talk about my previous week in the hospital.

"She has small cell cancer in her lungs," my mom said. "Grandma doesn't know what that means, but I figure cancer is cancer—not good. Do you know anything about it?"

Her words hit me hard. Gina, one of the first patients I cared for during my internal medicine rotation, had been diagnosed with small cell lung cancer. I flashed back to the somber conversation between the attending physician and Gina about the grim prognosis. Small cell lung cancer was uniformly fatal. Most deaths occurred less than a year after the initial diagnosis.

I wished I could have forgotten everything I knew about medicine—that I had never studied the pathology of lung cancer or that I had ever cared for a patient with small cell lung cancer. But I knew too much, and I could not escape the immediate, brutal truth: my grandma would probably be dead by this time next year.

"Jamie," my mom said, collecting her strength. "What do you know about it?"

I wanted to lie to her. I wanted to tell her that I was uncertain of the prognosis. But I also felt a responsibility to share what I knew, especially since the prognosis of small cell lung cancer was one of the more definite things in medicine. I think my mom could sense my hesitation.

"It's okay. I won't say anything to Grandma. Just tell it to me straight," my mom said. Then, putting on her nurse's hat, she said, "Healthcare professional to healthcare professional—what's the prognosis?"

Taking a deep breath, I told her that Grandma—her mom—would probably have less than a year to live and likely much less.

"That's what I thought," she responded, and I could hear her choking back tears.

"I've got to go, Mom," I lied. What I needed to do was find a place to have a good cry. We hung up, and I started walking, unconcerned where I was going as long as it was away from people. After some haphazard turns down seemingly endless corridors, I stumbled upon the hospital library. I decided that the stacks of books provided as good a hiding place as any. I sat on the floor and drew my knees to my chest. The tears came with a force I had never experienced before.

———

A half-hour later, back on rounds, the supervising resident pulled me aside.

"Are you okay?" he asked, noticing my bloodshot eyes.

"Not really," I said, unsure whether to reveal the news about my grandmother. "But, I'll be fine."

"I won't pry, but you don't look fine," he responded. "If you need to take a little time for yourself today, just let me know. I promise you don't have to worry about your grade or anything like that."

During the past few days, I had grown to trust the supervising resident and his judgment, so I blurted out what had happened.

"I just found out that my grandma has small cell lung cancer."

He cast his eyes downward. Everyone in medicine—regardless of whether he ultimately became a pediatrician or a plastic surgeon—knew that small cell lung cancer was an indisputable death sentence.

"Why don't you go home? Don't worry about coming in the rest of the week," he said. "Really, it's no problem. Go. Now."

Part of me wanted to, but part of me also didn't want to risk taking the time off. I didn't want to process everything in the seclusion of my apartment. I thought it would be better to be around people, even if they were people I had only known for a few weeks.

"No, I'll stay," I decided.

As the day ended, I grew nervous. I realized that I needed to call my grandma—something I had been dreading all afternoon. Thinking back to my mom's earlier suggestion, I returned to the one place in the hospital where I could do nothing other than smile: the nursery window. Standing there, gazing in at the tiny, squirming babies, I dialed my grandma's number. She answered the phone in the same way she always did whenever I called.

"Oh, Jamie, it's you!"

"Gram, you wouldn't believe where I am right now."

"Where?" she asked, playfully. She seemed like her normal self.

"I'm standing outside the newborn nursery looking at all the beautiful new babies."

She giggled.

"I remember when you were born. How happy Grandpa and I were! We drove right down to see you and—oh, my—weren't you the cutest little guy?" she said. "But, boy, were you a crier. I'd never heard a baby cry so much as you did those first few days. You turned out okay, though."

Then, without skipping a beat, she changed the subject.

"Did your mom tell you about my doctor's appointment today?"

"Yes."

"Well, I've got so many of those good memories stored away. And I'm going need them. The doctor said it's not good at all."

"I know."

I heard a clicking noise on the other end of the line.

"Jamie, someone else is calling. It might be my doctor. I have to pick it up. I'll talk to you later. I love you."

"I love you, too, Grandma."

The phone went silent. I pressed my face against the nursery window and began to weep quietly.

Chapter Eighteen

Seizure

DURING THE NEXT SEVERAL DAYS, my grandma's health continued to deteriorate. We found out my grandmother needed hospice care and soon—the disease had already spread throughout her lungs. She was left with little time to do anything other than put her things in order and say the things she needed to say. With the drop of a hat, I knew I might have to place my pediatrics rotation on hold and fly home to say good-bye. But for the time being, I welcomed the distraction of the hospital.

My supervising resident, who seemed surprised by my continued presence in the hospital, decided to assign a new patient to me, one who didn't appear very sick. Each time I passed the patient's room, I watched his mother as she angled a bottle of formula into the mouth of the insatiable child. By anyone's approximation, the pudgy folds of the child's belly signaled that he received adequate care and nutrition. On all accounts, he was fine—except that a week earlier, he had suffered a severe seizure after being fed diluted formula. Fortunately, the condition was reversible, and it would not result in any long-term disability. Still, our medical team was concerned about the child's well-being.

The supervising resident insisted this patient would provide a good opportunity for me to learn about the social welfare system (meaning none of the other residents wanted the frustration of spending hours on the phone with government social welfare employees). I also imagined the supervising resident didn't think I was in the best mental state with everything going on at home. This was an easier patient for me to follow.

—•—

Shanti Sainte, a thirty-year-old who functioned at the level of a mature fifteen-year-old, had little support in place to raise her son. Although her mild mental disability had pushed her to the fringes of society, she still functioned independently, and she managed to keep a low-income job and maintain a small apartment. Aside from some help from her older sister, she did not receive any other form of financial or physical assistance. In part, the social welfare system had abandoned her, and in part, she had avoided help. I discovered that the social welfare system had taken Shanti away from her own mentally disabled mother. When Shanti delivered her first child, she went about raising him to the best of her abilities—alone.

As I developed a rapport with Shanti over the ensuing days, I began to understand how the whole situation had unfolded. When her son developed a slight temperature a week earlier, she made the logical assumption that his stomach might be upset. To reduce the stress on his stomach, she watered down his formula. A day later, when her son started to shake while lying in his crib, Shanti became concerned, and she walked him the four blocks to his primary care physician. Not for a moment did I suspect that any of her actions had been malicious. Still, however innocent her intentions, I couldn't ignore that she had endangered the life of her son.

I made some suggestions about finding help for Shanti and her son. Usually, Shanti reflexively responded, "I am a good mother. I take care of my baby." Having watched her over the preceding several days, I completely agreed—she had demonstrated equal, if not better, basic parenting skills when compared to many of the parents I had encountered in the children's hospital. Ashamed that I had implied anything to the contrary, I assured her that I understood, and I reframed my intentions.

"I want to find a way for you to get premixed formula," I said. "And maybe even someone to help you around the house."

"Oh, I see," Shanti said. She always ended our conversations by saying, "Well, okay then. You have a good day, sweetie."

Nevertheless, despite Shanti's warm smile, I could see distrust lurking behind her eyes.

I had a discouraging talk with a social worker, who told me that few resources were available to mentally disabled parents.

"Can I get her in home nursing care?"

"No."

"Can I write a letter of medical necessity for reduced utility bill fees?"

"No."

"Can I help get her child into a paid day care?"

"No."

Most assistance came from volunteers who would sporadically visit a home and teach basic parenting skills. Much less was available in the way of financial support or routine home care. Even the most basic goal of the medical team—to ensure that someone would check in on them once or twice after their return home—was impossible to arrange. Our team exhausted our list of possible ideas, except for one that had been suggested earlier, one that we fiercely resisted: filing a referral to child protective services (CPS).

It seemed paradoxical that the only way to secure support for a child and his mother was by declaring the mother negligent, or abusive, or both. Yet, doing so would guarantee a follow-up by a state-appointed social worker, who would then evaluate the living situation and help arrange any required interventions. Of course, a CPS referral carried overwhelmingly negative connotations. In the same way families resist labeling a dying loved one as "do not resuscitate" out of fear of receiving subpar care, I knew that a referral would stigmatize the mother as a bad parent. Mostly, I worried how Shanti would interpret the referral. She was already intensely distrustful of the healthcare and social welfare systems, and I feared we might scare her away once and for all. If that happened, it would be impossible to secure the resources Shanti needed to continue taking care of her son at home.

Unfortunately, our medical team did not have any other option. With much reluctance, I called in the CPS referral. While I spoke with the CPS social worker, I took great care to emphasize the point that we did not suspect child abuse or neglect in any way. Making the CPS referral chafed against everything I had been taught about doing no harm to patients. At a minimum, this would cause upset to an innocent mother, whom I considered as much my patient as her son. After hanging up the phone, I went to run damage control.

I attempted to explain to Shanti the rationale of filing a CPS referral. She nodded as she always did, but instead of speaking, her bottom lip just trembled. Every so often, I paused to assess if she had comprehended what I had said. She just continued to nod. When I finished, she spoke.

"I am a good mother. I take care of my baby," she said, tears rolling down her face. "Why are you gonna take him away from me?"

Shanti had heard exactly the message I feared she would hear: "We don't think you are an able parent who can provide a safe home." I assured her that she was doing the right things, and that we had no intention to take her son away from her. But it was clear that I had poisoned the bit of trust I had built up over the previous days. I felt defeated by the backward system, and I left the hospital that day seething.

The next morning, with great trepidation, I poked my head into Shanti's room. She glared at me. I tried to ignore the previous day's events and went about my normal morning routine. I pretended that everything was normal and unchanged. I couldn't bear thinking about the suffering I caused this good-hearted mother, who—if she had the proper resources and support—could create a living environment in which her child could thrive. Attempting to avoid her anger, I turned to leave the room, but my conscience got the better of me.

"I know you probably don't like me much right now," I said. "But I really do believe in you. I think you're a good mother who is doing all the right things. I want to see your son go home with you. I really do. That much I can promise."

I couldn't tell if Shanti believed me, but judging by her refusal to look at me, I thought probably not.

Finally, after a week of calling various social agencies, writing letters of medical necessity, and in the end, making that dreadful referral to CPS, the pieces began to fall into place. Although the CPS referral had initially provoked bad feelings for all of those involved, slowly everyone began to realize that this was less a case of child abuse and more a case of societal neglect.

Oddly enough, the system whose reputation consisted of taking children away from their parents ended up being the saving grace for Shanti and her son. A social worker assumed control of the case. She would follow the family during the immediate period following the discharge. Home-based teaching would be provided regarding safe feeding, bathing, and parenting techniques; counseling was arranged for the mother, and a generous supply of premixed formula was secured through a city-funded program. With this support, the medical team felt comfortable discharging the child home with his mother, and I felt confident that they would thrive. The supervising resident let me deliver the good news.

A warm smile spread across Shanti's face, and after she set her child in the crib, she flung her arms around me and squeezed tightly. Although I was grateful for the services provided by the child welfare system, I still felt unsettled that it required a formal referral to CPS (the last place on earth where any scared parent would go to look for help) to secure the basic support that should have existed in the first place. While that was a sad social commentary, nothing could distract me from noticing the smile on Shanti's face when I told her she could take her son home.

Chapter Nineteen

Indiscriminate Hands

A FTER THREE SHORT WEEKS on the inpatient pediatrics ward, I transitioned to the outpatient clinic. On my second day at the clinic, one of the pediatricians, Dr. Levitt, invited me to accompany her to court. A city judge had summoned her to testify in a child abuse case. Because the incident with Shanti and her son was so fresh in my mind, I thought this might provide a good lesson about a case of *true* child abuse. From what Dr. Levitt told me, unlike my recent brush with the child protection system, she was scheduled to testify against someone who really had committed a grave crime.

"All rise," said a booming voice.

Swarms of people moved back into the courtroom. A young man stood parallel to me, just a few feet closer to the judge's podium. We wore identical khakis, similar button downs, and the same serious expressions. In fact, only a mahogany railing separated us. With a few steps, I could have easily changed places with him. Those few feet of space troubled me—I knew that he would never have the option of stepping to the other side of the railing where people with hopes and dreams and viable futures sat watching.

A stodgy, old man stood next to the defendant, and he gazed repeatedly down at the yellow legal pad in his hands as if searching for a clue about how to proceed. I could see that the paper was sparsely covered with several lines of illegible script, which provided an indication that the lawyer probably would not find what he was looking for. It looked like he had carelessly scribbled those few sentences down on his way to the courtroom that morning.

Finally deciding on some combination of thoughts, the lawyer stood to address the court, and his lack of enthusiasm was apparent in the drone of his voice. Without knowing why the defendant was in the courtroom, anyone would have surmised that the defendant's lawyer did not believe his client's plea of innocence. Anticipating the lawyer's canned comments, the judge, known for her gruff, no-nonsense attitude, stopped the lawyer mid-sentence and requested that the defendant stand to address the court.

"You, Albert Green, the defendant, are being tried for the charge of child abuse. This charge is a felony in the Commonwealth of Pennsylvania, and if convicted, you could serve up to twenty-five years in prison. Do you understand these charges?"

Albert appeared visibly shaken. He responded that he did understand, and his voice quivered. While he spoke, I bit at my lip—the duration of the possible sentence far exceeded the defendant's young age. A few days earlier, when Dr. Levitt invited me to accompany her to court, I would have tossed aside any feelings of sympathy. After hearing Dr. Levitt recount the short version of what had happened, I developed a striking disgust for Albert, though I felt oddly unsettled harboring such powerful, negative emotions.

For most of my life up to that point, I could argue that I had never truly experienced hate. For me, the word held the same dirty connotations associated with other four-letter words. I used the term sparingly, and when I did, hate was still only something I thought I knew about from reading historical accounts of crimes against humanity. But I understood the moment I saw the evidence photographs. The Polaroid pictures displayed a bloody, puffy foot of flesh cocooned beneath layers of plaster and gauze. Standing there looking at the graphic photographs, I *felt* hate.

The sensation caught me by surprise. It oozed into my veins and coursed throughout my body. It boiled over. I clenched my fists and ground my teeth. Albert's hands had beaten without discrimination: he had broken his baby's leg, crushed his ribs, and bashed in his face. I hoped the child would never have to see his father again. I wanted to imagine Albert sitting behind bars in a small prison cell, miserable and remorseful about what he had done.

"Judge. Judge?" Albert said as most eyes in the courtroom focused on him, waiting to see how the judge would punish this unsolicited outburst. Before the judge could react, the young man teetered to the side. He slumped against his frail, unsteady lawyer, who provided even less in the way of physical support than he did legal. Caught off guard, the lawyer fell to the ground with a thump, followed soon after by the sound of his client's body crumpling onto the floor next to him.

In an entire courtroom full of people, only a single body sprang into action. In one fluid movement, Dr. Levitt—the same person who had cared for Albert's bloodied, beaten child and was to testify against Albert—hoisted herself over the mahogany railing and landed next to his body. Without hesitation, she instructed the court deputy to call an ambulance. She placed her ear close to her patient's mouth, listened for breathing, and with her hand across his neck, felt for a pulse. She found both. Within a few moments, Albert's eyes opened.

After a bit of questioning, the physician determined that Albert, because of his nerves, had not eaten breakfast that morning. She continued to ask him about his medical history, concerned that he might have some other underlying medical illness. All the while, she held his hand, primarily to monitor his pulse, but also to provide reassurance—the young man had probably fainted from the sheer fright of his bleak future. Dr. Levitt made it known in those brief moments that he was not alone—not every person in that courtroom hated him.

It would have been hard to tell otherwise. Aside from the young man lying on the ground, the rest of the courtroom carried on with surprising normalcy. The judge retired to her chambers, the district attorney used the time to study her notes, and the courtroom audience turned their discussion to the latest tabloid news. The court deputy rolled in a tray of food and soda for the judge and lawyers, slowing only to maneuver the cart around Albert's body, and then he made his way toward the judge's chambers. Albert's own lawyer sat in a chair shaking his head as if he had just endured some grave injustice. Under his breath, he affirmed to himself that he would file a claim for any physical damages he incurred.

As people busily tended to their own needs, Dr. Levitt waited—without success—for someone to bring Albert a glass of cold water. No one had thought to offer him a can of soda or a glass of juice. In fact, once the defendant had opened his eyes, no one appeared to think much of anything about the young man. Blatant contempt replaced the fleeting sympathy he had commanded during his moments as a patient. Finally, a glass of water and a damp towel appeared. Dr. Levitt dabbed Albert's forehead and continued to monitor his pulse, and they waited for the ambulance to arrive.

Throughout the rest of the day, I experienced a profound sadness—not simply for the abandoned defendant, nor solely for the grave injustice of a beaten baby, but sadness because of the realization that humanity could not seem to straddle those two extremes. A rare few can care for both an abused child and the abusing parent. The attitudes apparent in the courtroom, from the stark indifference of the court to my own inability to reconcile my emotions, verified that most of us struggle to acknowledge that people who abuse children require as much help as the children they hurt. Still, there are those special few who touch the world with unprejudiced hands, who can stroke the foreheads of both a black-and-blue baby *and* a collapsed child abuser. Like Dr. Levitt, those people have indiscriminate hands and unconditionally accepting hearts.

CHAPTER TWENTY

TEACH BY EXAMPLE

"UH-HMGGM."

After the attending pediatrician, Dr. Bleerfetter, swallowed his gigantic bite of food, he caustically addressed me.

"Yes?"

A drop of oily dressing from his sandwich hung at the corner of his mouth, fell onto his pressed white coat, and left a greasy trail. I introduced myself as the new medical student who would be working in the outpatient pediatric clinic for the next several weeks. I had to repeat this process every day with a new attending physician, because there were so many pediatricians in the practice and each one only worked a half-day per week. Dr. Bleerfetter didn't note my name, nor did he look my way—he was completely focused on devouring his roast beef sandwich.

"I saw the new patient. Should I present the case to you while you eat?"

"Uh-hmggm."

I took this as a yes and began to present the medical history of the child I had just examined.

"He's a four-year-old obese boy with a history of controlled asthma whose mother brought him to the office because she is worried about his loud, nighttime snoring."

I looked up. Dr. Bleerfetter was still gulping down his sandwich, and it appeared that if he wasn't careful, he might choke himself.

"On exam, he has wheezes on forced expiration. Otherwise, his lungs sound normal. His tonsils are enlarged, but they don't completely obstruct his oropharynx. He also has redundant neck tissue."

While I waited for a response, the physician wiped the corner of his mouth, pondered my presentation for a few moments, and then responded.

"Sounds like the diagnosis is that he's fat."

Somehow, I had expected a slightly more thoughtful consideration of the boy's problems, especially coming from someone who didn't have the world's smallest belly. He motioned for me to follow and I trailed him into the exam room. I wondered how he planned to address and treat the diagnosis he had just made.

"Hi. Are you the mom?"

"Yes," she said, timidly holding out her hand.

Ignoring her outstretched hand, Dr. Bleerfetter walked to the sink where he proceeded to lather his hands. He kept his back to the mother the entire time. He cut right to the chase—he began to interrogate the mother, not once making eye contact.

"What do you feed him for dinner?"

"Well, he likes spaghetti a lot. Sometimes he'll eat grilled cheese sandwiches. Oh, and hot dogs," she answered, confused why she was being questioned about her son's diet. She had brought him in for treatment of his snoring.

"How many hot dogs do you make him for dinner?"

"Three or four," she responded.

"Three or four? No wonder he's got breathing problems—you're making him fat!"

I glanced at the young boy who promptly burst into tears. His mother appeared on the verge of tears, too.

"I am not fat! I am not fat!" the child said.

I was ashamed to be standing in the same room with this doctor, who had completely sabotaged any chance at forming a therapeutic relationship with the mother and her child. I remembered being back in the operating room with Dr. Greenwald, and how I had felt incapacitated by the authority that accompanies those who wear long white coats. I wanted to calm the mother and soothe her child, but I knew that if I tried to do that, I ran the risk of alienating the attending physician. And, like it or not, he was ultimately the one who graded me, not the mother. Like before, I had to swallow my desire to intervene. I tried to reason with myself: "A good grade will land me in a better position in the future, where I can effect change and stop these silly abuses of power." My justification didn't ease the sting much because in my heart of hearts, I knew I should stand up for the little boy, regardless of my grade.

Dr. Bleerfetter didn't notice my uneasiness and was completely oblivious to the mother's shock at his callous and damaging words. Looking down while he scribbled notes in the chart, he continued to probe the mother about her parenting style, and he took the opportunity to berate each of the choices she made in raising her son. He concluded with his bottom line.

"You're the reason your son is fat. You're the reason he is having trouble breathing. It's time you take some responsibility and take better care of him. No more hot dogs. No more grilled cheese. No more video games. No more soda. You got it?" Dr. Bleerfetter said, with the tone of an angry parent. "I expect that he will have lost five pounds by the next time I see him."

With that, we swooshed out of the room, never once having addressed the mother's concern about her son's snoring. As we left, the appalled mother reached for her young child, trying to calm his sobs and soothe his bruised self-image.

Outside, Dr. Bleerfetter debriefed me about the encounter, and then he insisted that he had a pearl of wisdom he wanted to share with me.

"You've got to learn that sometimes you need to take a stern stance with patients. Unless you come down on them hard—sometimes real hard—they'll never change," he explained.

While he talked, I found it impossible to look him in the eye. My gaze focused instead on the small drop of oil spreading outward across the lapel of Dr. Bleerfetter's long white coat.

———

That afternoon, I paired up with a different attending physician. I avoided the fat, oily man I worked with that morning. Less than an hour after the scarring encounter with the young asthma patient and his mother, I visited with another young, obese boy who had identical symptoms. In a similar manner, his mother described how she had grown concerned while listening to her son gasp and gurgle at night. After I had finished taking a detailed history, including the all-important information about the boy's diet and exercise (a high-calorie diet filled with fatty foods, snacks, and sodas, and not enough exercise), and then completed a physical exam, I stepped out of the room and gave an encore performance of the morning's presentation to the new, different attending physician. She nodded and focused on the young boy's story.

"How many hours of television does he watch per day?" she asked. "You said he doesn't get enough exercise. Is his neighborhood safe enough for him to spend time outside? Some of my families live in dangerous parts of the city, and even if they wanted to, it would be unsafe for the children to play outside. We'll have to investigate some more."

Then we went back into the young patient's room together.

"Hi, guys!" the attending physician said, greeting the mother and the son as if she had known them for years.

"So what's your name?" she asked the young boy, keen on making his acquaintance before proceeding any further.

"Jake," he replied, and then spelled it out for her, "J-A-K-E."

"Nice to meet you, J-A-K-E." She laughed.

After introducing herself, the physician verified the history I had gathered, and she listened intently as the mother offered her own assessment of her son's problem. Then, the physician smiled and turned to her young patient.

"So, I hear that you've been having some trouble breathing at night, Jake?"

He looked at his mother for reassurance, and she urged him to answer the physician. With a quizzical look on his face, he shrugged his shoulders.

"Do you know if you snore?"

He smiled shyly and cast his playful gaze downward. Then he looked up and giggled.

"Yes. I think I make noises like my dad does," he said in a matter-of-fact voice. He looked at his mom the entire time for support. We all laughed.

"Do you want to make the noises go away?" the physician asked.

"Yes," he said, giggling.

"Well, then I think I can help," she said. Even though the initial medical management consisted of the same interventions that the gruff physician had recommended to his patient earlier in the day, she approached Jake and his mother using a much different tactic.

"Do you think you and your mom can do two things for me before I see you the next time?"

"Yes."

"The first—every time you play your video games, I want you to spend the same amount of time doing something outside. So, if you play twenty minutes of video games, then you should go and ride your bike or play with your friends for twenty minutes."

"That sounds like a fair deal, right Jake?" his mother asked. "You can do that, right?"

"Yes, I can do that," Jake said as if the doctor had just charged him with an important, grown-up task.

"The second—and I'll need your mom's help for this one—I'd like you to drink no more than one diet soda a day. The rest of the time, either water or skim milk. This one may be harder, but it's just as important. Do you think you can do this?"

"Yes," Jake replied, while his mother nodded along.

"Good! So the next time I see you, I'm going to ask you how you've been doing with both of these things. Okay? And I'm also going to ask if you still are making sounds like your dad!"

Jake found her last comment tremendously funny, and he erupted into uncontrollable giggles of pure delight—the kind of infectious joy I've only ever witnessed in children.

"I'm gonna tell my dad what you said about him," Jake cackled, in between his shivers of laugher.

With that, we walked out of the room. Outside the door, the attending physician gave me some advice.

"Did you see how I turned my goals for weight loss into a fun task? I usually find that this works the best, especially since his mother can now use the same tactic. The other thing I like to do is keep the goals simple—only one or two easy ones at first. Then, once those things become second nature, I move on to another."

I was captivated by the attending physician's simple, yet powerful wisdom. Once she finished, I looked her straight in the eye and thanked her for the lesson.

"You're welcome," she said, turning on her heels and opening her next patient's exam room door. From outside the room, I could hear her good-natured greeting.

"Hi, guys!"

I stood next to the door and waited. I knew that I would soon hear the giggles of a child as the physician introduced herself to her new, little patient.

Chapter Twenty-One

Comfort Amid Chaos

DURING MY FINAL WEEK of the outpatient pediatric rotation, I had the opportunity to experience a side of pediatrics that most people didn't know existed: pediatric hospice. As part of a home visit program, medical students could accompany a nurse to visit the home of a chronically ill child to gain a better understanding of what life was like outside the hospital. When given the choice of several different patients, I opted to visit a pediatric oncology patient. I thought it might give me some insight into my own grandmother's current struggle with cancer.

As we entered the patient's house, the stench of stale air assaulted me. These kinds of smells weren't supposed to linger anywhere except inside the halls of nursing homes, and certainly not in the home of a dying child. I had expected something different—more like the clean dignity of the sleek hospital rooms to which I was accustomed. The only reminder of anything remotely hospital-like was the young girl's bed, around which everything else in the cramped row house seemed to orbit—piles of junk, heaps of clothes, empty plates, and discarded food wrappers all radiated outward from the nucleus of her bed. Much like a forensic detective, I could recreate the recent activities of her family members using the locations of the various objects, and one thing was definite: now, her family lived, breathed, and probably existed solely to take care of her.

The hospice nurse and I both moved toward the center of the room, and I tried to ignore the smell that I associated with impending death. The journey was not without hazard: I bumped into a collection of empty oxygen tanks, which were arranged like bowling pins directly inside the doorway. The heavy metal cylinders clattered against the floor and crunched the discarded medication boxes beneath them. More carefully this time, I navigated the piles of clothing, plates, and cartons, and advanced toward the young girl, whom I discovered was neatly tucked into her bed despite the surrounding clutter.

During my car ride with the hospice nurse named Frannie, she recounted her first experience with Ally, the cancer patient, several weeks earlier when she had been asked to become involved with Ally and her family.

"At first, Ally's situation did not seem so hopeless. She was receiving chemotherapy, and she was fighting the fight. In the hospital, everything was controlled. But during her hospitalization, I watched as she lost each of her bodily functions," Frannie said with an even voice. "It became clear that she would die within a short time. That's when her family insisted on taking her home to die in her own bed."

I didn't understand how Frannie did her job. Although clearly invested in providing exceptional care to her patients, she told me about Ally's tragic story without as much as a tear. Meanwhile, I sat with wet eyes and looked out the car window.

"Once her family decided they wanted to move her home, they re-directed their efforts to make it happen. Everything was focused on getting her home. I tried to help them understand what it meant—that they would have a lot of new responsibilities."

She paused for a moment.

"Ally's parents and her brothers are amazing," Frannie said. "Amazing."

I waited for her to tell me why.

"They knew exactly how much work it would take to get Ally home. And how much more it would affect their lives to have her die in their home," she said. "And they refused to have it any other way."

———

For someone just barely acclimated to the controlled environment of death in a hospital (the only place where I had ever been exposed to death), the chaos of the family's home shocked me. The first thought that crossed my mind was, "How the hell did we let this happen?"

Everything was much more complicated here. Ally's brother had to carry her limp body upstairs to use the bathroom. Her mother had to reschedule shifts at a low-paying job so that should Ally miraculously open her eyes, she would see a familiar face. Her father had to coordinate schedules with delivery of the almost daily shipments of oxygen tanks and pills. Amid all these responsibilities, the waves of clutter and disorder had engulfed everything but the pristinely maintained hospital bed.

Under the direction of Ally's mother, I safely navigated the remainder of the space between the front door and the girl's bed. Once beside her, I realized that the smell I had initially thought to be the odor of death was anything but that—Ally exuded the scents of baby powder and fresh linen. The other odor emanated from everything else that had been pushed aside—things that could be ignored to focus on Ally.

In the moments that followed, I did the only thing I knew how to do: I laid my hands on top of Ally's hands. Her skin was soft and warm and slick from just-applied moisturizer. Ally's mother nodded preemptively as Frannie discussed the well-known medical plan: under the guidance of the hospital doctors, Frannie would continue to increase the morphine doses to curtail Ally's pain and ease her labored breathing. She would use larger, more humane doses that might relax a weary, suffering body.

As we retreated toward the door, Ally's family remained clustered in close orbit around her bed. I no longer noticed the odor or the clutter. Like her family, I was completely focused on the slight, fragile figure lying at the center of their world. Ally's mother resumed her afternoon routine of combing her daughter's hair out straight before tying it into braids. Her brother continued to whisper lines from Ally's favorite books into her ear. Her father fell asleep on a couch tucked into the corner of the room in an attempt to save enough energy to sustain him through another all-night watch.

My initial reservation about enabling this young girl to die at home was replaced with a different thought: "Is the hospital the best place for a child to die?" Today, my intuition told me that Ally's family had made the right choice. Even amid the smell, the grime, and the seeming chaos, Ally's family had found peace and order in their tireless quest to remain firmly joined together. For the short time they could, they remained united in their humble, well lived-in home.

Several days later, I got a call from my mother—the call I had dreaded for the past few weeks.

"Jamie, it's time to come say good-bye," she said, her voice choked with tears.

I crumpled under the weight of those words, but somehow I felt less anxious imagining my grandmother's last days. If she were as comfortable as Ally had been when I visited her in her home, I knew that my grandmother would be in a loving, safe place, surrounded by her family. Then somehow, I knew that I would find the strength to hold her soft, wrinkled hand and tell her one last time, "I love you."

PSYCHIATRY

Chapter Twenty-two

Kryptonite

I DUCKED OUT of the rain and into the old, decrepit building on the corner of Ninth Street. The fourth floor housed one of the city's locked, inpatient psychiatric units where I was to spend the next eight weeks learning how to care for mentally ill patients. True to form, the building captured the familiar institutional look of Hollywood psychiatric facilities—the tiled walls and matching linoleum floor appeared borrowed from the set of *Rain Man*.

The stormy day outside added to the eeriness of the building's interior, and by the time I reached the actual entrance to the psychiatric ward, I felt as if I had crossed into a different world. I nervously pushed a buzzer beside the hefty metal door and waited.

Within seconds, a pair of bulging eyes pressed against the Plexiglas porthole in the door and scanned my face with an intensity that I had never before experienced. Despite the barrier between us, I gasped and stepped backward, frightened by the unyielding stare. A few moments later, the face jerked away from the small window, and I realized that a police officer had yanked the man back into the recesses of the unit. The officer re-approached the entrance and buzzed the door open, and I used the weight of my entire body to move the heavy steel door.

"Welcome to the *Twilight Zone*," the officer muttered under his breath.

A small lounge was to my left. An old black and white television blared from the corner of the room. A dozen or so people sat watching a program with their painfully empty eyes focused on the grainy screen.

"Don't you look at me that way! Take your eyes off me!"

I realized the yelling came from one of the patients, who—gravely offended by the sitcom—screamed insults back at the television. Someone else hummed a discordant tune, and another patient rocked back and forth in his seat. Still shaken from my encounter just moments earlier, I felt uncomfortable. Luckily, the psychiatric resident behind the staff counter noticed my flustered expression and my short white coat, and ushered me into the familiar safety of the physician's workroom.

She told me that the psychiatric ER had been busy the previous night, and the team had six new patients to admit to the ward. Overwhelmed with things to do, the resident introduced me to the unit staff, gave me a brief introduction on admitting a psychiatric patient to the hospital, and then thrust a new patient chart at me, all within five minutes.

"Here. Edward Jacobs was 302'd for walking into traffic on the interstate. He tried to see if he could fly by jumping off the highway divider. Get a history."

Almost as an afterthought, she reminded me to plan an escape route before talking with Edward, and then she sent me on my way to interview him. Before I left the workroom, I sheepishly inquired what "302'd" meant.

"Committed by police," she responded.

Over the noise of the television, I called out Edward's name, and a thin, disheveled man leaped from his chair. The pair of probing eyes I'd seen earlier belonged to my new patient.

I led Edward to a small interview room. As he passed by me, the unmistakable scent of an unwashed body wafted by me. The tiny space quickly filled with the potent stench, and I silently questioned how long he had gone without a shower. Judging by the clothes he wore, I assumed he had lived on the street for a long time. He wore layers of shirts, and his pants were stained from sleeping on dirty city sidewalks. I breathed through my mouth to avoid the smell, and I wondered how fast I could finish the interview and escape to fresh air.

True to the information contained on the 302 form, Edward had a large abrasion on his arms from his crash landing on the rough highway pavement. I took a deep breath—Edward really had stopped traffic on the freeway while attempting to fly. Somehow, I had expected to walk in and discover that he had a reasonable explanation. Never having worked before with psychiatric patients, I found it difficult to believe that someone might be motivated by an alternate reality. His oozing, bloody arms reinforced that I knew nothing about Edward's world.

He chose to occupy a seat that backed up against the only wall in the room without a window or a door. His eyes danced from place to place, and they scanned the contents of the room with the same intensity as when he had evaluated my face through the front door. His facial expressions changed rapidly, alternating between unprovoked giggles and pensive stares, and I wondered what motivated his behavior. During those silent first moments, I began to realize that Edward responded to cues that I could not see or understand. After he satisfied his curiosity regarding his whereabouts, Edward began the conversation.

"You know who I am? I'll give you a hint. I can run faster than a cheetah and faster than a silver bullet. I have six girlfriends," he said in one breath. "You figure it out yet?"

"I'm Superman," he said, unable to wait any longer for my response. "I can swim faster than sharks. That's why I have so many girlfriends. Did you just see what I did with my eyes? I can see through you."

With these few sentences, Edward had allowed me to look into his mind. He revealed the scattered ideas that raced through his head, and in some context, probably made sense to him. His tangential stream of thought left me feeling disjointed, and I wondered what I could possibly say in response to his outburst. How does one address a patient who has just proclaimed he is Superman? Earlier in the workroom, my resident had hastily instructed me to address patients in the same way that they referred to themselves, so I took her advice and followed Edward's cue.

"It's nice to meet you, Superman. You've told me about some of your powers, so let's talk some more about why you're here today," I said. "Why do you think you're here?"

Edward looked at me, and in a strange way, I felt that he actually might be looking through me. As I waited for a response, I wondered if he could see the frightened thoughts running through my head. Then, without shifting his intrusive gaze, he responded.

"Who sent you to ask that? What do you know? Did I tell you who I am?"

Edward talked profusely for the better part of the next twenty minutes. Although at times I attempted to direct the conversation so I could obtain his medical history, he clearly had control of the meeting. His mind raced with so many different topics that my head spun while listening to him.

After the half hour passed, I ended the conversation to give Edward a break. After he left the room, I tried to piece together what little history he had given me. I found it impossible to make sense of his story. And why hadn't he mentioned his experience on the highway?

That afternoon, I discussed Edward's treatment plan with the psychiatry resident. Together, we identified that the man was schizophrenic and would likely benefit from treatment with an antipsychotic drug.

I wondered what the effect would be on Edward. Would a medication help calm the thoughts in his head? Would he ever interact normally with other people? Or did our conversation together reflect something inflexible, something hardwired in his brain? It intrigued me to think that he might gain some touch with reality. I put the pharmacy order into the computer and felt oddly guilty by the prospect of tinkering with a person's reality.

It eased my mind when the medication did not transform Edward into a different person overnight. For the next several days, we continued to meet in the small interview room for thirty minutes at a time, and we discussed whatever occupied Edward's mind. While the calming effect of the medication made him less labile when he talked, the content of his thoughts remained the same. He still referred to himself as Superman, and he still believed that he could see into my mind.

Like that first day, many of the next days were spent trying to piece together the fragments of life that Edward described with such zeal during our sessions. I had also been able to contact Edward's parents, who told me more about his childhood, although the new information did not help make any more sense of Edward's thoughts. His parents had lost touch with their son after he had started living on the street several years earlier.

By the fourth week of my rotation, Edward's disordered pattern of thinking had become so normal to me that I found it abnormal when he started to hold conversations that were more logical during our daily meetings. His appearance was the first indication that something had changed. One by one, Edward replaced his smelly, layered shirts with laundered button-downs that his parents brought him. On his own volition, Edward showered and shaved each morning, and then he combed his hair with a neat, slick part right down the center. Most striking, however, were the lucid conversations that Edward began to take part in and sometimes initiate. He surprised me one day when he asked if I felt prepared for an approaching exam, indicating that he had retained a portion of the prior day's conversation.

The medication that I had initially regarded with caution transformed Edward from an unkempt, acutely psychotic man into a person who could communicate more clearly and interact with the world around him. I found it incredibly rewarding to watch Edward walk down the hall of the psychiatric ward and laugh with other residents as they joked about the horrible french toast served in the cafeteria.

In the medical hospital, many of the therapies for sick patients could only temporarily slow down the progression of their diseases—like Alden, who we had put on beta-blockers to stall the development of heart failure, or Gina, whom I recently learned had undergone palliative chemotherapy for her lung cancer. In Edward's case, I believed that the intervention had placed his life back on a course destined for normalcy. So long as he took his medication, he could live a life based in reality. How could anyone not desire that?

Instead of discharging Edward to the routine pathways of halfway houses or city shelters, Edward went home with his caring parents, who beamed to have the son that they knew back. Before sending the trio off, the attending psychiatrist sat down with the parents to discuss Edward's diagnosis of schizophrenia and answer any questions they might have.

In particular, the attending physician stressed the importance of recognizing that Edward's illness would be a lifetime process, and that it would require a healthy tolerance for the ups and downs. I think that the warning was equally directed toward me, but it fell on deaf ears. I was completely focused on watching Edward walk out of a psychiatric ward with his parents. It seemed we had discovered Edward's kryptonite—he hadn't mentioned Superman in days.

CHAPTER TWENTY-THREE

TRUTH OR DARE

"You know those moments right before a thunderstorm breaks? When the clouds open up, and the air courses with static electricity? It feels like that."

The on-call psychiatrist was describing the phenomenon that occurs right before a busy night in the psychiatric ER. She had promised me that during at least one of my psychiatric ER shifts, I would experience the feeling for myself.

Frankly, I had begun to doubt her—my first two shifts had passed quietly and without incident. The first night, we watched over several intoxicated patients who needed a place to sleep off their drunkenness, and we refilled medications for another patient who had run out of her mood stabilizer medications. The second night, we admitted a severely depressed, grieving, elderly man to the inpatient unit.

By the time I arrived at the entrance of the psychiatric ER to begin my third shift, I had the foreboding sense that tonight would be different, just as the attending physician had described. In fact, outside the locked entrance to the ER, a line of people had formed as if they were standing in line for a concert. In a process similar to the locked inpatient unit, after I flashed my badge through a small Plexiglas window embedded in the door, a uniformed security guard buzzed me in. I passed the row of waiting patients, feeling as though I had a backstage pass to an event. The security guard acted like a bouncer—I watched him deny and push back some of the people closest to the entrance.

I focused my eyes straight ahead and walked down the corridor to the glass-windowed control room. From this protected space, the nurses and physicians could observe each patient's room. The place was packed. Even the tiny waiting room, which was usually empty, overflowed with patients.

"Oh good! You're here," said the attending physician as she bustled back into the room. "It's nuts here tonight—no pun intended. I told you, didn't I?"

"It's exactly as you described," I replied.

"If you don't mind, take Ray with you, and go get a history from the guy sitting in the small office next to the waiting room. I didn't know where else to put him. Every other room is full."

Ray was one of the male nurses who worked in the psychiatric ER. I imagined that while filling out a job application, he had specified that he possessed the largest pair of biceps known to humanity. He uniformly had a calming effect on patients, even the rowdiest of them.

Ray and I headed down the hallway toward the small office where the patient, a male about my age, waited. Realizing that the room could not comfortably hold the three of us, and wary of leaving me alone with the patient, Ray coolly suggested that I leave the door open to prevent the office from becoming too stuffy. The patient nodded. Ray wedged himself in the doorway behind me. I sat down and began to talk.

"So what brings you to the ER tonight?"

"The police. That's what. The fucking pigs," he said, his biting tone catching me by surprise. "I was with my buddies earlier tonight, partying, because it was one of their birthdays. We went to the bar to have a few drinks. Man, was that fun. I like beer all right, but tonight we were celebrating, so we hit the scotch. I can hold my alcohol damn well—I was outdoing all of them. Then I suggested that we should go dancing in the city, and everyone told me how great an idea that was. So we got in my car and headed out. While we were driving, this cocky cab driver decided that he wanted to race me, the fucker. He should have known that I'm a goddamn amazing driver. I could take on Mario Andretti, that's how good I am."

I fully expected him to pause for a breath since up until this point, he had talked without pause, but he somehow managed to continue.

"The asshole cut me off and I crashed into a guardrail. You know, out by River Drive. That's where. The cops showed up and told me they needed to take me in. I told 'em I was fine, just a little happy from my scotch, but nothing I couldn't handle. I told them I would just jog home, since I'm a triathlete, but they wouldn't listen. So the fuckers brought me here. I'll get their asses. I'm a friend of the mayor, you know. People know my name."

"I'm sure they do," I thought. "Probably from reading it so often in the public ledger."

Although I had only spent a short time in the world of psychiatry, I felt confident the man suffered from bipolar disorder. He had all the classic symptoms of a manic episode: pressured speech, grandiosity, decreased need for sleep, and increased energy.

"Do you take any medications?" I said, slyly attempting to confirm my provisionary diagnosis.

"Yes. I sometimes take Depakote. But I haven't been using it lately. I don't think I really need it. I couldn't figure out why they made me take it in the first place."

I finished the interview and rose to leave the room. The patient looked up at me angrily.

"You gotta get me out of here soon. I've got things to do. If you don't, I'll sic the mayor on both you and those fucking cops. Got it?"

"Sure. Got it," I said, imagining the scene he would create once he learned the police had committed him to a minimum of seventy-two hours in the locked inpatient unit. But at the same time, I couldn't ignore that he was in dire need of psychiatric attention.

———

The remainder of the night passed in a similarly crazed manner. I cared for a succession of patients, each of whom seemed crazier than the last—and, it was impossible to differentiate the patients who might harm me from those who were not dangerous.

Not long after I had interviewed that first young man, I talked with a shifty-eyed male who claimed to be suicidal. He insisted we admit him to the hospital immediately, or he would kill himself. While he waited for us to make our determination, he laughed and joked with his friends. His threats seemed out of character with his mental state, which struck both the attending physician and me as suspicious. With additional follow-up questioning, the man confessed that he was, in fact, a member of the Mafia who needed a temporary place to hide.

Soon after, I met another patient who had walked herself to the psychiatric ER because she thought she might shoot her neighbor if she did not get some help soon. For a full hour, she described her raging emotions and scared me in the process. Afterward, she asked for a sandwich and a soda—we provided these to patients once they'd been evaluated. Shortly after she'd eaten, she insisted we discharge her from the ER, and she vehemently denied she'd ever uttered a word about harming her neighbor.

My final patient of the night frightened me the most. Despite Ray's superhuman strength, it required three of us—Ray, the attending physician, and me—to restrain the acutely agitated man. While he thrashed, kicked, and attempted to bite anything in his vicinity, he screamed, "I'm gonna fucking kill you all, you fucking spies!" Once Ray had successfully restrained the man, he plunged a needle full of a tranquilizer into his shoulder. During the course of the next several minutes, the yelling diminished until the patient dozed off.

By the end of the evening, I didn't know what to make of any of this or whom I could believe. All through the night, patients had been telling me stories, but I couldn't tell what was true and what was not. Each time that I thought I had uncovered the *real* truth, a patient would throw another kink in his story, making me less trusting of his words.

It was difficult not to develop a cynical attitude while working in the psychiatric ER. I felt as if the patients were constantly playing me for a fool and using my goodwill to fulfill their own needs—whether for a meal or a place to hide from a "Mafia boss." Granted, many of the people did require some form of psychiatric help, but I still found it incredibly challenging to discern those people from the actors.

The most important reason to maintain a healthy dose of cynicism was for the sake of safety—I had to be alert all the time, expecting the worst in people, to protect myself from harm. The moment I let my guard down, someone like the kicking and screaming psychotic man might take advantage of the situation and hurt me, if for no other reason than that, somewhere in his mind, he thought it might be a good idea. But finding that compromise between respecting a patient's reality and maintaining my own sanity and safety required far more experience than a few, short shifts in the psychiatric ER. As I left the building that evening, I thought about the attending physician. She had dedicated her life to finding balance among a bunch of mentally unstable people.

On my way out, she called to me from behind her desk.

"You wouldn't believe it. I just got off the phone with the assistant to the mayor. He politely asked me to expedite the transfer of that bipolar patient to a private facility and to keep it quiet. Apparently he's the son of a well-to-do family, and they don't want this leaking out." She had a look of amazement on her face. After letting the information sink in for a few moments, we both burst into incredulous laughter. He'd proven us wrong—he really had kept his word and called the mayor.

CHAPTER TWENTY-FOUR

CONVERSION

"I'M NOT REALLY sure. Everything stops, and then I don't remember anything else until I feel my dad shaking me awake."

That's how Anna Himmel, the sixteen-year-old patient, had described the blackouts she'd experienced during the course of the preceding several months. Both Anna and her father had recounted the same history. At no particular time and for no particular reason, Anna would suddenly stare off into space immediately before her body would slump over. She never stopped breathing, nor did she have any visible seizures. She appeared as if she were sleeping.

Previously, Anna had always been sitting or lying down when one of her attacks came over her—she was never injured. Recently, the spells had become more frequent and more severe, and Anna had fallen during gym class, banging her head and bruising her shoulder. After this occurred, her father decided to bring her to the hospital.

For the first several days of her hospital admission, Anna underwent every test in the book. The cardiologists worked her up for a possible cardiac origin of her fainting episodes. The neurologists observed her brain waves during one of the spells to rule out a seizure disorder. The infectious disease doctors looked for a possible infectious cause of the girl's symptoms. The metabolic doctors studied her family tree for rare genetic disorders. Everyone came up empty-handed.

After each of the doctors from the different specialties had retreated in defeat, Anna's primary medical team called in the pinch hitter: the psychiatrist. During the previous nine months, and in particular, during the last several weeks spent on my psychiatry rotation, I had witnessed firsthand the bad rap that psychiatrists got—they were often referred to as "pretend" doctors who practiced the equivalent of voodoo medicine.

Although I had subscribed to that belief in the past, my recent experience with the psychiatric world had begun to teach me otherwise. Having watched Edward respond to his antipsychotic medication, I started to believe that we knew more about the brain than I initially imagined. Nevertheless, once I had heard Anna's story, I did not think that the psychiatry team would have any real insights to offer. Anna didn't have any symptoms of depression, psychosis, or—as far as I knew—any other classifiable psychiatric disorder. Furthermore, if she did have a psychiatric condition, I couldn't figure out how to link it to her fainting spells.

It surprised me when the psychiatrist confidently diagnosed Anna with something she called "conversion disorder." While she explained it to me, I stared at her in disbelief. The meaning of conversion disorder was exactly how it sounded: the body "converted" stressful mental events into physical symptoms—a short circuit between the brain and the body. The psychiatrist attributed Anna's spells to the recent stress of her parents' divorce. When Anna could no longer handle the strain, her body put itself to sleep.

This particular ailment—conversion disorder—caused me a significant amount of my own mental pain. I found it much easier to understand a disease process for which I knew the underlying physiologic cause. If a patient's creatinine level went up, he had renal failure. If I heard a harsh heart murmur radiating to the neck, she had aortic stenosis. With disorders of the mind, I had a more difficult time accepting the presumed, yet unproven explanations. In some way, it made sense that Anna could turn off her scary thoughts and instead do something far more palatable: sleep. Still, without any biological proof, it required a great leap of faith to believe in the validity of this diagnosis.

I could not, however, ignore that after a bit more investigation, it turned out that Anna's spells coordinated perfectly with the times that she experienced acute stress: after she had moved away from her mother who lived in South Carolina, after her parents had finalized their divorce, and after her father had begun dating a new woman. The temporal relationship did beg at least some attention. Since the additional tests continued to come back negative, the medical team followed the psychiatrist's recommendations, and we called in a psychologist to talk Anna through her problems. We hoped that by talking about her feelings, her body would naturally correct the short circuit, and the blackouts would cease.

I found the "hoping" part wholly unsatisfying, especially after seeing several psychiatric patients respond to appropriate medications. Unfortunately, in Anna's case, since we had no understanding of her disorder, we had no medicine to offer her— we just hoped for the best. It felt similar to the way that patients with fatal diseases sometimes believed in novel therapies unproven to have any efficacy in humans. Although the consequences were different, it still seemed as if the medical community had failed Anna. She was no better off after the sharpest minds had considered her puzzling symptoms.

—

By the end of my eight-week psychiatric rotation, Edward's case remained the most memorable recovery I had witnessed. In fact, I viewed his improvement as the most significant response to medical therapy that I had observed during the course of my entire year. In my eyes, he was one of the few who made it to the other side of illness without too great a scar.

Every once in a while, I found myself imagining what Edward might be doing. Was he rebuilding his relationship with his parents? Had he found a job? Had he enrolled at a local community college? Since his discharge from the psychiatric ward, I had developed high ideals for his life, much in the way I imagined a parent did for his growing child, and I found great satisfaction in considering the possibilities.

Continuing to question that golden advice that "common things are common," I chose to ignore the most probable outcome, the one that my attending physician had so carefully pointed out during Edward's family meeting: most people with Edward's illness face lifetimes of constant struggle with medications, their minds, and their relationships. My brief time on the psychiatric ward had left me only with momentary snapshots of patients' lives. I did not have the opportunity to experience the repeat admissions and chronic issues associated with mental illness.

Five weeks after finishing my psychiatry clerkship, I went for one of my usual jogs through the museum district of the city. Every day around rush hour, a large van pulled up to one of the curbs, and local church members dished out warm food to the park's homeless residents. As I jogged past the long line of people on that cool, spring evening, I locked eyes with one of the men, and I stopped dead in my tracks.

Beneath re-accumulated street stubble and wisps of long, greasy hair, I recognized the unmistakable face of my first psychiatric patient. Edward stared directly at me—or perhaps through me—and then quickly shifted his gaze. I wondered if he'd recognized my face. A split-second later I realized he had. As I looked behind me, I noticed that Edward had left his place in the line to follow me. Had he remembered me as one of his old doctors? Or had he incorporated my face into one of his alternate realities? Either way, I understood that he did not welcome my presence.

"Hey man! What the fuck? Don't look at me. Do you know who I am? Who I am!"

That was as much of the conversation as I stayed to hear. I picked up my pace and sprinted away from the commotion. Out of breath, I continued to run until I had found the anonymity and safety of the crowded city streets.

I now had answers to some of my questions, although the answers did not match up with the lofty expectations I had created in my mind. As I imagined, Edward did move out of his parents' house, but instead back on to the street and into a life devoid of medication or mental healthcare. I realized how cavalier I had been to think that Edward would adhere to the plan we outlined at his hospital discharge. Of course, he would struggle with relapses of his illness! Of course, he would have issues with medication compliance! I realized that Edward had been far more perceptive than I had ever imagined. He *had* seen right through me. He knew better than I that from the moment we met, I had nothing more than a temporary treatment to offer him. I wondered if, in his mind, he viewed his return to the street as a success. After all, Edward—better known in his world as Superman—had just survived his battle with kryptonite.

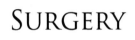

SURGERY

CHAPTER TWENTY-FIVE

STAT

"**WHAT TIME SHOULD I SHOW** up tomorrow morning?" I asked my new supervising resident on the phone, fully expecting him to respond, "Seven AM for rounds." After all, I didn't know any of the patients, which led me to believe that I probably wouldn't be very useful before rounds on my first day.

"Five," he replied.

"No, better make that four thirty," he said, correcting himself. "It's going to be a busy day tomorrow."

I gulped. Four thirty AM? What could possibly require anyone to wake up that early, let alone a superfluous third year medical student?

Before I could say anything else, I heard a click, and then the buzzing tone of a dead line. He hung up on me. No, "I look forward to meeting you." No, "Good-bye." No nothing. He just hung up. The interaction made my stomach churn. Although my classmates had told me that I should develop a hard shell—and fast—the interaction with my new supervising resident made this idea painfully real.

The following morning, after riding my bike down the center lane of the deserted city streets at 3:30 AM (I had decided to plan in some extra wiggle room that morning, just in case), I reached the hospital only to find that every entrance was locked shut until 6:00 AM. Never before had I arrived at the hospital at this ungodly hour, so I hadn't anticipated that it would require special access to get inside.

With my anxiety building, I jogged around the perimeter of the hospital to see if I could locate the ER, where I knew I would almost certainly find someone to buzz me in. Eventually, I did find the entrance, and someone did let me in. But once inside, I encountered the same problem all over again—the individual wards also had restricted access during the early morning hours.

It took me another half hour to find a janitor who, after some strong convincing and pleading on my part, agreed to let me into the surgical intensive care unit where my supervising resident had instructed me to meet the team. With not a minute to spare, I located the small residents' room and opened the door.

No one was there.

For an hour, I sat behind the desk wondering if I should page the supervising resident. If I did, there was a good chance I might needlessly annoy him, especially if he was catching a rare moment of sleep or doing something else important. But if I didn't page him and I missed rounds, I ran the equal risk of establishing myself as an incompetent fool. By this point in the year, I had realized that first impressions *did* matter.

Fortunately, I didn't have to wait for too much longer. Right around 5:30 AM, the team shuffled in one by one. They all appeared to have come from their homes. Each person took off his winter jacket and replaced it with a long white coat. I wondered what I had missed. Why had I needed to show up at 4:30 AM?

"You the new med student?" said one of the more bleary-eyed residents. "That's my seat," he muttered, pointing his finger at my chair. "Out."

With my nervous energy from starting a new, unfamiliar rotation, I leaped from the chair as if someone had hit an eject button. I wanted to start on the right foot with my new team.

"I'm sorry," I said.

The resident who had ousted me from my seat took his position behind the small desk in the room, and I assumed that he was my new supervising resident.

"We decided late last night to start rounds a bit later today," he said, offering a roundabout, halfhearted apology for making me wait.

"No big deal," I responded, and I honestly meant it—by this point in my training, I had come to fully embrace the "oh shit" theory that Dr. Brixton had explained to me months ago. I knew that these first few days with the new surgical team would be unsettling, but that I'd nevertheless get through it. It would be easier if I didn't knock myself into a tailspin. So I didn't.

"I'm Jamie, by the way," I said, holding out my hand.

No one shook it. In fact, I don't think that anyone noticed my extended hand. Their attention turned to "running the numbers," and it took me right back to earlier in the year when I had worked with Dr. Greenwald. The lowest ranking team member—me—would show up extra early to collect and record each patient's laboratory values, urine and stool output, body temperature, blood pressure, heart rate, and respiratory rate, and then regurgitate the results to the rest of the team during rounds.

For the next twenty minutes, I watched as the supervising resident berated, belittled, and scolded his interns for letting an aberrant lab value slip by unchecked, or for not ordering labs in the first place. In less than a half hour, I understood that the next two months would test the limits of my tolerance. If I could survive this, then I could survive the remainder of medical school—if I still wanted to be a doctor by the end of it all.

After we finished reviewing the patients' lab values, everyone rose in unison and filed into the hallway. The resident who had taken the most grief from the supervising resident looked at me with apologetic eyes, and then he shoved a plastic bedpan stuffed with medical supplies into my hands—the treasured "scut bucket," as my classmates had lovingly referred to it. Although I'd heard an awful lot about the scut bucket, I imagined that I would at least have the dignity of carrying an actual bucket, not a glorified bedpan. Before I could make any additional inferences about the bedpan and its relationship to my role on the team, I noticed everyone had disappeared down the hallway.

Standing next to the first patient's bed, the sympathetic resident quietly directed me under his breath on how to unroll the gauze, or how much saline to squeeze on the bandage, or how long to cut the pieces of tape—a crash course in the intricacies of scut bucket duty. I tried to follow his instructions, but the pace was too fast. Once I had figured out how to open the package of gauze, the supervising resident was already yelling for tape. By the time I found the tape, I think smoke was pouring out of his ears.

It didn't take me long to realize that surgeons demanded perfection. Surgeons expected pristine lab values from their patients, infallible performance from their residents, and expert all-around bandaging skills from their medical students. As the prime example, the supervising resident seemed to regard everything—even the little things—as high-stakes endeavors, as if someone's life might depend on whether I cut the bandage thirty-one millimeters long, instead of thirty millimeters.

A few minutes later, while we huddled around another patient's bed and examined a wound, a blaring overhead speaker disrupted everyone's concentration.

"Code blue team to room four hundred, stat! Code blue team to room four hundred, stat!"

The air grew tense. Code blue meant that someone in the hospital needed immediate medical attention, usually because of a heart attack or some other life-threatening condition. Each resident stopped what he was doing and took off in full stride down the hospital corridor. The helpful resident grabbed me by the collar of my short white coat and pulled me in the direction of room four hundred. As we approached the room, I remembered its inhabitant: a young woman with cystic fibrosis, whom we had examined just minutes before.

When we had visited with her, I felt extremely vulnerable to see someone so close to my own age so sick. Now I stood at the fringe of the group, not sure how to reconcile my fear of interacting with her and my desire to help her. In the end, I opted to remain in the background, scared by her situation, and subsequently, by my own mortality.

Other members of the code blue team began cardiopulmonary resuscitation (CPR). Someone stood at the head of the bed trying to insert a breathing tube down the girl's throat, while someone else loomed over her limp body and pressed down with his full body weight. Each time he completed a chest compression, I exhaled, temporarily spared from the horrendous sound of ribs cracking and the awful sight of the girl's body heaving from the brutal force required to keep her blood flowing.

The supervising resident stood near the girl's bed and directed the entire ordeal. "You—send a blood gas! You—get ready to take over compressions. Someone call the operating room and tell them to prep for an emergency thoracotomy," he yelled. "And someone else page the attending surgeon, stat!"

With astounding calmness, the supervising resident simultaneously directed the resuscitation efforts, interpreted the girl's lab values, attempted to diagnose what had precipitated the situation, and coordinated the transfer of the girl to an operating room. In that moment, I realized why the supervising resident had demanded perfection from his team members: he had but a few seconds to make life-and-death decisions, which left him no room for error.

"She's got a massive pulmonary embolism," he decided. "Go, go, go!"

And they were off, wheeling the patient down the hallway toward the operating room while a resident, perched atop the gurney, continued chest compressions.

Trailing behind the mass of medical personnel, I found my way to the operating room, somehow managed to scrub and gown, and then installed myself, again, at the periphery of the group. From the sidelines, I watched as the supervising resident and the attending surgeon, who had arrived in a hurry, heaved the girl onto the operating table. Without the usual preparations for surgery, the supervising resident swiped a knife across the girl's lifeless chest. Then, the angry growl of a bone saw drowned out the commotion, and the surgeons cut down through the young girl's sternum.

Once they exposed her heart, they worked furiously to isolate the pulmonary vessels, which they suspected housed the clot that had caused her condition. After a few minutes, they filleted open one of the large pulmonary arteries and found a sizeable plug of congealed blood. With a pair of forceps, the supervising resident pried the clot from the vessel. As it came out, I noticed that the stringy clot was as wide as my thumb—it had blocked *any* blood from flowing between the girl's heart and her lungs.

Even though they removed the clot and sewed the vessel back together, the young girl's heart refused to start. She lay naked and exposed on the operating table, and her body bucked unnaturally each time the surgeons tried to shock her heart awake. Still, after several minutes of unsuccessful attempts, no one wanted to give up the resuscitation effort. A shared thought was apparent on their faces: "She's too young. If only I continue for a bit longer, just maybe." But the young girl's body would not have it. Five minutes later, after a resigned nod from the attending surgeon, the supervising resident surrendered to reality and abandoned his efforts.

"Time of death is seven fourteen AM," the supervising resident noted quietly, and then he began sewing her chest back together. Before he did, he asked the nurse to cover the girl's body with several blankets to give her some privacy, and he took a few extra moments to arrange the blankets carefully over her small body. Even though the girl was dead, his primary concern was to preserve her dignity.

I noticed that my body was shaking uncontrollably—the kind of teeth-chattering, unable-to-catch-my-breath shiver that I'd only ever experienced during a hard cry. I'd just witnessed my first death, and—most unsettling—it had been the death of someone my own age. During the past year, several of my elderly patients had died. But in each case, I had arrived at the hospital only to learn that my patient had been transferred to the intensive care unit where he had "expired," as the ICU doctors put it. Most of these discoveries had taken place while I stood in front of a computer screen and scrolled through a patient's electronic record only to see the boldface notation: DECEASED. That's how I discovered the death of my first patient. As much as her "virtual" death had hurt, I recovered quickly, buffered by the computer from the actual experience of death. But standing there in the operating room with a lifeless young body, especially one whom I had seen living and breathing just minutes before—it knocked the wind out of me. I couldn't keep from imagining my younger brother lying there on the cold steel table.

Once the supervising resident finished making the girl's body presentable for her parents, the cadre of doctors and nurses filed out of the operating room. Dejected and depressed, none of us spoke a word. I knew we were all thinking the same thing: "This could have been my niece or my daughter or my sister." Yet, it wasn't. So we continued as best as we could with the business of the day.

We returned to the bedside of the patient we had abandoned to respond to the code call. The supervising resident reassumed his uncompromising position.

"No, cut that gauze shorter!" he barked. "Why didn't anyone order calcium levels last night? Pick up the pace, med student. We don't have all day!"

I might have continued to mistake his harsh words as a personal attack (as I had only an hour earlier), had I not just witnessed the young girl's death. Although I knew that the length of a piece of gauze probably would *not* make the difference between life and death, I now understood the importance of treating if as if it might—it promoted a sense of respect for the incredible trust that a patient places in the hands of his surgeon. Recalling how the supervising resident had so carefully covered the body of the young girl, I cut the gauze to the correct length and draped it flawlessly across the patient's healing incision.

"Satisfactory, but still too long," the supervising resident reprimanded me as we moved on toward the next patient's room.

"Now tell me," he said to the team. "Why didn't this patient's blood get drawn yesterday for an albumin level?"

We all stared blankly at the papers in our hands.

"That's unacceptable," he said.

Somehow I understood that there would always be something more to be done or something else to improve on, and as long as there was, the supervising resident would do everything in his power to remind us that we were all intimately responsible for the lives and deaths of our patients.

Chapter Twenty-six

Her Voice Alone

DURING THE EARLY MORNING HOURS of my first overnight surgical call, a flurry of white coats broke the still of the room belonging to one of the team's new patients. A succession of commands set hands into motion, and the supervising resident worked quickly to assess the elderly woman's labored breathing.

I stood watching as Ellie Cropp lay in the frightening darkness, probably much like she did as a child. Her frail, bony fingers were white as they clasped the rails of her bed. Her eyes were wide open, and she stared straight up at the ceiling. I heard her pray for the commotion to end.

"Please let me die. No more of this," she moaned. But by the time anyone realized she had spoken, the numbers on the monitor had stabilized, and the surgeons exited the room as hurriedly as they had arrived.

The frequent interventions became a daily routine for Ellie and the surgical team. But with each subsequent encounter, I grew increasingly worried. Ellie would whimper defeat into the darkness while her doctors made decision after decision.

"Another chest tube!"

"Please don't," she pleaded.

"Let's bronch her."

"No," she moaned.

"She needs an operation."

While I was familiar with the "do everything possible" attitude of medicine (I had witnessed internists prescribe drug after drug for a suffering patient or gynecology-oncology surgeons administer just one more dose of chemotherapy), the brutal nature of surgical procedures forced me to confront the idea of pushing relentlessly onward. The attending surgeon attempted to subdue my anxiety.

"She's demented. It's okay. We're making the right decisions along with her family," he said. He sounded like he didn't have the patience to engage me in a moral discussion.

Late one afternoon, I went back to visit Ellie. While she lay in her hospital bed and stared at the ceiling, I sat down in a chair beside her and began to read her hospital chart. I discovered that she had mesothelioma, a rare and deadly lung cancer probably caused by the asbestos dust that her husband had carried home on his work clothes. She'd raised three children who lived in the area, and her husband had passed away several years before. In the back of the chart, I found a simple, hand-typed statement making known her wish for a peaceful ending.

My eyes shifted back to Ellie. I felt terribly uneasy. She lay there alone, tangled in tubes and wires, and waited for her fate.

Each day during rounds, I silently questioned the list of new orders: Did she need to go to the operating room again? Was another procedure truly in her best interest? Where was Ellie's voice in all of this? The more I thought about her final request, the more I wondered why no family conference had occurred. Someone should have sat with the family to clarify Ellie's idea of a gentle ending. Instead, her peaceful petition remained tucked in the back of her chart.

I visited Ellie again, and I noticed her lips moving under the hissing oxygen mask. As I lifted the mask from her face, Ellie mumbled the same words as she did every day.

"Let me die."

I touched her shoulder, and swayed by the party line I had grown accustomed to, I found myself ready to reply, "Your new chest tube is going to help with the pain." But Ellie continued to speak.

"Call my daughter," she instructed, and then she rattled off a phone number.

<hr />

That same afternoon, after working up the nerve to address the team about something other than Ellie's laboratory values (which, up until that point, was the only reason I had license to speak), I timidly voiced Ellie's wishes during rounds.

"Ellie asked if we would contact her daughter for her," I said. "It sounded very important."

I handed the daughter's phone number to the attending physician, and I hoped that this might result in us discussing Ellie's typed wishes. The supervising resident compared the unfamiliar digits with those in his notes.

"This is a nonsense number," he scoffed.

Immediately, I felt my face flush over and my ears grow warm. After the team dispersed, I sat quietly in the empty residents' room, and I felt embarrassed for having questioned the surgeons' intentions. I now had proof that Ellie suffered from dementia, and I wondered if I had read too far into the legitimacy of her pleas.

I met Ellie less than a week after witnessing the death of the young cystic fibrosis patient, and I found it difficult to determine where to draw the line. No one, including me, had wanted to stop the rescue efforts for the girl. The surgeons had performed a gory, emergency procedure known to have a minimal chance of success, and I probably would have done the same.

Yet, confronted with Ellie's situation, I felt myself resisting and questioning every attempt to prolong her dwindling time in this world. At first, I wondered how I could be so morbid to think about denying Ellie any life-saving procedures. Soon, though, I realized that it wasn't that I wished for her death, but that I wanted to minimize her suffering and preserve her dignity. How much care was enough? In my mind, I could not reconcile the two situations to arrive at a hard-and-fast rule. The answer, of course, lay somewhere in the back of Ellie's chart, somewhere in the conversations that she'd had with her children, and somewhere in the way her family had watched her live her life. Nevertheless, the question remained too painful for anyone, including the medical staff, to consider. Ellie's voice continued to go unheard beneath the roar of her blowing oxygen mask.

During her final days, no one knew for sure what kind of end-of-life care Ellie desired, and no one accepted the difficult responsibility of finding out. Her family made decisions from afar without visiting or talking to her. Her physicians replaced difficult bedside conversations with convenient calls for procedure consents. Not even I—someone who had initially believed her nonsensical ramblings—continued to pay much heed to Ellie, who lay there demented, but also surprisingly consistent in her pleas for peace.

The morning after Ellie died, I sat in the cafeteria and stared out the window into the blackness of the predawn hour. Ellie's family had made it in time to say good-bye before she passed away, and I found some relief in knowing that. After a few moments, my thoughts turned inward. Although I knew that I had ultimately failed to protect Ellie's voice, the situation forced me to begin asking myself the hard questions—the kind of questions to which I knew there were no sufficient answers. In the process, maybe I had given Ellie's voice volume, not as much as either of us hoped, but it was a start.

CHAPTER TWENTY-SEVEN

CONTROL

"AFTER MY THIRD TRIP to the bathroom, I decided I'd just leave. You don't know what it's like to be a forty-year-old man and shit your pants. It was my first and last date in years," Avery said, glancing at me with a half-laughing and half-loathing look in his eye. "The chicks don't dig that."

"I'm sorry, Avery," I said. I didn't know how to respond. "That sounds awful."

I realized that I should have left it at "I'm sorry."

"I'm sorry, again," I said.

"It's okay," he responded. "I'm just glad to see a familiar face. You'll be at the surgery looking out for me, right? Keep me safe from those doctors?"

"Definitely," I said, and I found it amusing that he didn't consider me one of them. He'd obviously been entangled with the medical system long enough to know what the length of my coat signified.

About a month after I had begun my internal medicine clerkship, back at the beginning of my third year, I had first met Avery

Klein. He had come to the hospital for what he called an "IBD flare." Realizing that I had no idea what that meant, Avery took the opportunity to educate me in living color about inflammatory bowel disease (IBD), and in particular, ulcerative colitis—the specific illness from which he suffered.

Ulcerative colitis had caused Avery's colon to fill with millions of ulcers (much like canker sores of the mouth) that resulted in frequent bouts of uncontrollable, painful, bloody diarrhea. Although I had been taught to recognize the physical manifestations of ulcerative colitis, I had received little training about the accompanying psychosocial issues. That's where Avery came in. He had been quick to point out that more than he hated diarrhea, he hated his disease for the limits it set on his social life.

In detail, Avery had outlined for me the steps he took during one of his flares. The steps generally entailed stopping everything he was doing at work or at home, checking himself into the hospital, taking massive amounts of steroids—much higher than his normal, between-flares dosage—and returning home a week or two later, tired and depressed, hoping that he hadn't lost his job during the interim.

His visits to the hospital were no vacation. He spent most of his days either making trips to the bathroom (sometimes up to ten times an hour) to poop blood, or having grown tired of the constant back-and-forth, just sitting in the bathroom for hours, afraid to leave the safety of his toilet. Mostly, though, Avery hated the effects of the steroids. Over time, Avery had developed a sizeable potbelly, a plump face, and purple stretch marks across his arms, legs, and abdomen.

"Look at me," he said. "I'm a fat, middle-aged man, who eats a healthier diet than pretty much anyone out there. My diet consists of three servings of oatmeal a day—the blandest, most boring food known to man. It's the only thing that doesn't send me running to the bathroom, and yet these steroids make it look like I eat hamburgers and fries fifteen times a day. It's no wonder I can't get a date. Go figure."

I couldn't blame him for being angry. I would have been, too.

———

That afternoon during rounds, I learned that Avery had met with Dr. Ross, one of the attending surgeons who had undergone special training in bowel surgery. Dr. Ross specialized in performing an operation called a "total colectomy and J-pouch," which meant that after the surgeon removed a patient's diseased colon, he would fashion a makeshift rectum from the remaining small intestine. This pseudo-rectum allowed a patient to hold his bowels in a much more predictable manner and for longer periods, at least until he could make it to the bathroom.

Although Avery avoided surgery at all costs, thinking that it could only make things worse, he recently had started to consider the possibility. During a routine colonoscopy, Dr. Ross discovered several precancerous lesions in Avery's colon (a common finding in patients with ulcerative colitis). Avery changed his decision without hesitation: he wanted the operation, and he wanted it immediately.

Fortunately, Dr. Ross was happy to add Avery to his operating room schedule. He was the kind of physician with a tireless work ethic and a humbling dedication to his patients. In the several days that I'd spent with him, I'd watched him arrive at 6:00 AM each morning to round, begin surgery promptly by 8:00 AM, work right through lunch, and then round again in the evening. Most days, he didn't leave the hospital before dark, and although he frequently stayed later than that, he never complained or grew short with his residents.

Honestly, I couldn't understand how Dr. Ross did it—missing another dinner with his family, adding on an operation at the expense of the precious half hour he had set aside for a jog, or depriving himself of the opportunity to sleep in late just once in a while. He had relinquished all control of his non-hospital life to perform surgery. This seemed unfathomable to me, but was a godsend to patients like Avery. Dr. Ross scheduled Avery's surgery for the following day.

———

I met Avery in the preoperative holding area to say good morning before the anesthesiologist put him to sleep. Avery had a reserved, yet unmistakable grin across his face.

"I feel good, Jamie," he said. "Like I'm making the right choice. I won't miss my colon a bit."

"That's got to be a good feeling," I replied.

"Can I ask you one favor?" he said, slyly. "Will you make sure to give it the middle finger for me?"

We both laughed nervously.

Twenty minutes later, Dr. Ross made the initial incision down Avery's abdomen. I stood at the edge of the table, held a pair of retractors, and waited for Dr. Ross to expose Avery's colon. He cut down through the layers of Avery's abdomen, first parting the muscle and fat, and then he pushed aside the glistening, yellow intestines to reveal the back wall of the abdominal cavity. With sharp scissors, he carefully uncovered Avery's colon.

From the outside, the colon looked less threatening than I had expected. For the most part, it looked similar to the remainder of his bowel, just a little less flexible. In a series of several deft maneuvers, Dr. Ross tied off the colon at either end, freed the remainder of it from its resting place, and then, with two snips of his heavy scissors, hoisted the entire colon out of Avery's abdomen and onto a nearby specimen tray.

The colon landed on the specimen tray, and the friable tissue crumbled apart and oozed blood and stool. Before sending the colon to the pathologist, Dr. Ross called me over to the specimen tray. While I stood beside him, he carefully sliced open the remainder of the colon. The bowel wall—normally pink and smooth—looked like a cobblestone road. Blood seeped out from every crevice of the hideous tissue, and I understood the origin of Avery's frequent, bloody stools. Only then did I realize the true extent of how Avery must have felt about his diseased colon.

"Good-bye and good riddance," I whispered, adjusting the edge of my surgical cap with my middle finger.

After the surgical resident and I wheeled Avery to the recovery room, we rejoined the tireless attending surgeon as he began his next operation of the day: a gastric bypass. The patient, whom I had met the previous evening, weighed three hundred pounds. Dr. Ross reassured me, however, that she lived an incredibly healthy lifestyle, and much like Avery, had been dealt an unfortunate genetic hand.

Doreen Bell had attempted every diet in the book and walked as much as her knees could tolerate. No matter how hard she tried, she could not lose a significant amount of weight. Recently, the excessive weight began to catch up with her. She had developed excruciating back pain, her knees were beginning to give out, and most concerning both to her and Dr. Ross, the extra weight put her at tremendous risk for a heart attack. Doreen's mother had died at the age of forty-nine from a heart attack, and as Doreen approached forty, she understood that she needed to seek medical attention.

As she lay there on the operating table, I was struck by the surgeon's unfaltering assurance to everyone in the room that this surgery held the key to Doreen's health. Maybe I had seen too many tabloid reports of the miracle gastric bypass gone badly. But from what I'd read in the scientific literature, death was a real possibility. Nevertheless, I tempered my skepticism with the knowledge that Dr. Ross did have many years of experience.

The surgery went smoothly and without incident. Then, as nine pairs of hands plus mine lifted the woman's body from the operating table back to the gurney, I experienced the physical stress that her body was subjected to on a daily basis, and I hoped that the surgery would be the path to her success.

———

An hour or so after we had finished Doreen's bypass, I accompanied the surgical resident to perform a postoperative check, which consisted of reviewing Doreen's vital signs, ensuring that she had adequate pain control, and verifying that she was making urine. Despite passing the postoperative check on all fronts, Doreen still looked like hell. Her face was puffy from the anesthesia, and although the morphine seemed to control her pain as long as she remained still, whenever she moved, she groaned.

"Are you okay?" I asked.

"Ugggh. I feel awful, honey," she said. Then, with a half-smile on her face, she refuted her last comment. "But I'll be damned if I'm not going to lose my first ten pounds by my birthday in a month. It's my present to myself."

I felt certain that she would.

A few beds down, Avery was also recovering, and he looked similarly miserable—but he still had an impish grin on his face.

"Hey, man. Did you give my colon the middle finger?"

"Well, kind of," I explained.

"That's good enough for me," he said. "Thanks."

"My pleasure."

"I figure I've got a couple weeks of bathroom-free rest and relaxation in the hospital to catch up on my life," he said. "Then, I've been thinking, it's time to call that girl back—the one I ditched at the restaurant. Maybe with my new bionic pouch I'll be able to sit through a dinner with her."

Inspired by Doreen and Avery's unfaltering hope, even while in terrible pain following their life-altering (maybe even life-saving) operations, I realized the answer to the question I had asked myself a few days earlier: "How on earth did Dr. Ross keep such a demanding schedule?" By relinquishing some control in his own life, Dr. Ross had given both Doreen and Avery something that I too often took for granted—he had given them back control of their lives.

Chapter Twenty-eight

Indifference

B Y THE END of the second week of my general surgery rotation, I spent most of my time in the operating room, instead of just helping interns complete the daytime scut work on the wards. As much as I had initially enjoyed watching surgery and learning about anatomy firsthand, after a few surgeries, the experience grew tiresome—mostly because the surgeries lasted so long and my bladder was so small. But there were also the relentless jobs of holding the retractor blade (as I had initially learned to do back during my obstetrics rotation), or sucking up the exhaust of the Bovie with the suction catheter. Combined with my perpetual exhaustion, the tedium of standing for hours as a wallflower in the operating room did not make for an enjoyable experience.

One afternoon, as I leaned against the cold, steel railing of the operating table for the fourth consecutive hour, I looked up at the clock and hoped to discover that hours—not minutes— had passed. Displeased with the position of the clock's hands, I turned my attention back to the operating table in front of me. My eyes fixed on a tiny square of flesh surrounded by green drapes, the only reminder in the entire room that a patient lay somewhere among us.

"Closing time—three forty PM."

The voice of the attending surgeon, Dr. Ingblatt, broke my trance. She announced that we had finished ahead of schedule, and she decided to reward both the resident and me with the holy grail of surgical students: the opportunity to "close." After just a few surgeries, I had learned to dread that five-letter word. It meant that I had the particularly inglorious job—even less fun than standing in one position for four hours—of cutting the long tails off suture stitches. It also meant I would undoubtedly be scolded again for making the ends "too short" or "too long," despite the "perfect" length the day before. Silently, I resented the attending surgeon for what she was about to put me through.

As I shifted into suture-cutting position, I felt the painful tingle of blood flowing back into the stagnant parts of my body, and it jolted my senses awake. Apparently, the resident standing across from me did not experience the same second wind of energy—her eyes looked as tired as my body had felt while I stood watching the clock. If I appeared unenthusiastic to cut the sutures, then she looked twice as unhappy to sew the stitches.

Wary of her sudden responsibility, the resident's hands shook nervously as she attempted to pick up the patient's skin with her tweezers and make her first stitch. She fumbled with the instruments, and she poked the tip of the suture needle repeatedly into the patient's flesh, afraid to commit to any one pass of the needle. Even though the senior surgeons often left closing to the lower level residents, they still expected perfection. I sighed, resigned that the process would take longer than it should. My legs would have to tolerate another hour's worth of standing.

The majority of the hour passed quickly, although not for the right reasons. Each time the resident threaded a length of suture through the patient's skin, I had to jerk my head backward to avoid the wide, haphazard arc of her needle-wielding hand. Several times, she nearly sutured my hand directly to the patient's abdomen—that's when I began to realize the attending surgeon had given the resident too much responsibility. In most circumstances, this teaching method usually served its purpose, but in this case, I likened the resident to a soldier who had been handed a lethal weapon with minimal training.

While the resident unpackaged another suture, I let out a sigh of relief, thankful for a temporary respite. No sooner had I relaxed, than I felt a prick as the suture needle sunk into the flesh of my right index finger. The sharp, glistening half-circle of steel had effortlessly bitten through both layers of my double-gloved hand. I felt silly for having thought a second layer of latex would provide extra safety.

An overwhelming heat spread throughout my body. A deafening roar filled my ears. But these sensations soon gave way to the sickening, heart-pounding realization of what had just occurred. The resident looked directly at me, and I could see the terror in her eyes. At a loss for words, she said nothing. I didn't know if the needle had punctured the patient's skin before entering mine, and judging by the expression on the resident's face, neither did she. For the first time in my tenure as a medical student, I spoke out of turn and with authority rather than question.

"I got stuck," I said, stating the obvious. "I'm going to scrub out and go get help."

With an amazing calm, I backed away from the operating table, stripped myself of my surgical attire, and briskly walked out of the operating room in the direction of the occupational health office. After a short wait, a physician ushered me into the quiet of his examining room, and I began to recount the events of the preceding twenty minutes. I shook with worry the entire time. As soon as the words "suture needle" exited my mouth, far before I finished my story, the physician interrupted me.

"The risk of a puncture from a solid needle is minimal compared to that of a hollow hypodermic syringe," he said, matter-of-factly. Truthfully, had I sat in his position, I probably would have offered the same advice—the risk of infection from a solid needle stick was exceedingly low, especially given the circumstances surrounding the exposure. Nevertheless, despite my fright, he continued to spew numbers and statistics to mount a defense for what I understood would be his bottom line: "A case such as this does not require anti-retroviral prophylaxis." Almost as an afterthought, he promised me that he would have the patient tested for hepatitis and HIV, and that he would inform me of the results the following day.

Even though I wanted to believe his indisputable scientific evidence, in my irrational and emotional state, I wanted a prescription for prophylactic anti-retroviral medication. I knew of at least a dozen residents who had written themselves prescriptions for anti-retroviral drugs following a questionable exposure to blood or bodily fluids. As a medical student, I was in a vulnerable situation: I didn't have the ability to write my own scripts, and ever afraid of a damning evaluation from an instructor, I feared causing a scene by sticking up for myself. But sitting there with my own health on the line and realizing that no one else would look out for me, I found a sudden and surprising strength.

"I'm not leaving here without medication," I blurted out.

The physician looked up at me, and deciding that an argument would waste more of his time than it was worth, shrugged his shoulders indifferently.

"Okay," he said, and he took out his pad to write me a script for two doses of zidovudine—the same medication that pregnant HIV patients receive to prevent transmission of the deadly virus to their fetuses.

"In the meantime, just sit tight," he said, addressing my emotional state for the first time during our encounter, albeit in a roundabout way. "And try not to worry so much."

Easier said than done.

Dazed, I returned to my duties in the operating room, and I hoped no one had noticed my absence. In the middle of the next surgical case, as promised, the occupational health physician called Dr. Ingblatt to formally report the incident and request that Dr.

Ingblatt draw blood from the patient. As they conversed using the operating room's overhead speakerphone, I experienced—for the second time that day—the tingling feeling of shock while listening to Dr. Ingblatt's callous response.

"C'mon. That's ridiculous. He's just overreacting. We all have our first stick at some point," she barked in the direction of the speakerphone. She looked at me with glaring eyes. "It doesn't sound like it was a real one, anyway."

Three hours later, while the team visited the postoperative patients on rounds, I refused to look at the patient with whom I had become blood brothers. Before rounds, the surgical resident had tried to consent the man for an HIV test, but he had refused, unsure of why he needed testing for HIV. I wondered if it was because the surgical resident hadn't been able to admit to the man that she might have infected her student with his blood. The resident promised me that a senior resident would go back to consent the man after rounds. Despite the innocence behind the patient's refusal for HIV testing, I found myself angry and unable to stand in the same room with him.

Each aspect of the patient's life became part of mine, and even minute details knocked the wind out of me. His tattoo—had he contracted HIV from a dirty needle? His service in World War II—had he ever received a blood transfusion while wounded on the front lines? His recent foray into the elderly dating world—had he been aware of the increased rates of HIV infection in the elderly population? All of the possible unknowns were enough to drive anyone crazy. I felt even more scared because no one seemed concerned about drawing blood to find out the answers to my questions.

In the quiet of my apartment, my overactive mind sprang into action and plagued me into the twilight hours. Will my parents have to watch their son die from AIDS? Will it be a long, slow death? Morning rounds could not come soon enough, and when they did, I wanted to know one thing and one thing only. Did the patient with whom I had unwillingly become blood brothers have hepatitis or HIV?

Since no one mentioned the incident during rounds, I cornered the supervising resident directly afterward. He casually responded that after a busy night running back-and-forth between the emergency room and the operating room, he had forgotten to draw the patient's blood. He promised me he would get to it soon. I could not understand how anyone would treat my life with such disregard.

In the meantime, I had built up enough courage to go back to the patient's room to see if I collect some evidence myself. Perhaps I might gather some information about the man's risk factors. Much like I imagined the surgical resident had, I hid behind my white coat, afraid to make it too personal. I knew how bad I would have felt if someone had been stuck with my blood, and I didn't feel comfortable burdening the man with something that was out of his hands. Instead, I asked innocent questions about his tattoos and his time in the army to learn if he approached his life with cautious responsibility or with reckless carelessness.

The man smiled as he talked, and he provided me with entertaining—yet uninformative—stories about his past. Although the man opened up his life to me, I still resisted opening mine to him. I sat silently beside his bed and did not say a single word about why I was there. He seemed nice enough, and had I just said something, he probably would've consented to the test right away.

Later that day, once I found out that the supervising resident had obtained the man's permission for an HIV test, I wondered how the man would react the next time I saw him—now that he knew I'd been stuck with his blood. When we visited him on rounds that afternoon, I stood sheepishly toward the back of the group and attempted to remain as inconspicuous as possible. As the rest of the team finished changing his dressings, I walked out of the room to avoid any "You should have told me" looks from the man.

A few hours later, my pager vibrated against my hip, and it jolted me out of my daze. I dialed the flashing phone number on my pager.

"This is the Occupational Health Department," someone answered. I recognized the voice of the doctor who had counseled me about the needle stick.

"I'm returning a page for Jamie Feinstein," I said.

"Oh, yes. The results you were waiting for—they're all negative, son," he said, with a tinge of irritation in his voice. "Okay? Bye."

His uninterested attitude didn't matter—I felt instantly relieved as if I had a new lease on life. Oddly enough, my first instinct was to run directly to the patient's room and tell him that the test results had come back negative. But I stopped myself, realizing that I had never let this experience become *our* experience. In fact, everyone involved in the incident had kept the problem from becoming his own.

A few days later, I stood in my usual position and leaned against the cold, steel railing of the operating table for the fourth consecutive hour. I wanted to look up at the clock. Instead, although it took all my strength, I focused my attention on the operating table in front of me.

Call it a morbid exercise of the mind, but I tried my hardest to conjure up the fright I had experienced the days following the needle stick. I wanted to remind myself that the patient lying on the operating table had probably experienced similar fears right up until the moment he went to sleep. Even though, from a medical perspective, I knew a procedure like the removal of the gall bladder was routine and uncomplicated, I now realized that the patient had probably worried: "Will I make it through the surgery? Are my wife and children scared? Will I recognize my body afterward?"

Dr. Ingblatt's voice interrupted my thoughts.

"Closing time—two twenty PM."

On cue, I stepped into position. This time, I paid special attention to the length of the suture tails. When the patient awoke, I wanted him to see a neat row of perfectly trimmed stitches—a visible assurance that every aspect of his care had remained at the forefront of our minds the entire time.

CHAPTER TWENTY-NINE

THE KING AND I

AFTER COMPLETING MY GENERAL SURGERY rotation with the unfortunate experience of the needle stick, I was happy to move on to my subspecialty rotation. Not only did I escape the unfriendly work environment that Dr. Ingblatt had created for me, but the transition also meant that I was one-step closer to finishing the third year of medical school. Two more weeks with the vascular and cardiothoracic surgeons, followed by two weeks in the ER, and then I was done. The end was in sight.

Three days a week, Louie Brickfield sat on his throne, attached—literally—to the belly of a medical system by several feet of floppy plastic tubing as if someone had forgotten to snip his umbilical cord years ago. Without fail, every Monday, Wednesday, and Friday, the driver of the dialysis transport van would pull up to the curb of Louie's first floor city apartment and honk the horn. In response, Louie's frail figure would emerge from the apartment doorway. He would slowly hobble down the concrete sidewalk with his outstretched arms guiding the four-legged walker in front of him.

More often than not, Louie's feeble appearance elicited a friendly helping hand from a concerned passerby, but he uniformly rejected these offers as signs of weakness. On several occasions, the driver offered to spare Louie the inconvenience of walking and instead wheel him to the van using the portable wheelchair, but he had given up after Louie repeatedly refused his help.

By the time the van made it to the hospital, the staff of the dialysis unit would have his recliner waiting. The nurse would drape Louie's two colorful, homemade blankets over the back of the chair and lay that day's newspaper on the adjacent tray table. The staff followed this routine religiously—they knew that any deviation would result in one of Louie's famous fits of indignation. On a worn piece of paper taped to the counter of the nurses' station, several veteran staff members had scribbled a protocol of sorts that saved new nurses, physicians, and medical students from fumbling blindly through one of Louie's visits.

Nevertheless, many of those who survived the initial shock of his demanding behavior eventually developed a genuine desire to make Louie's difficult life a little easier. For just that reason, his longtime dialysis nurse still searched for ways, such as removing the jokers from his deck of playing cards, to draw out a rare smile.

My first encounter with Louie did not occur in the dialysis unit, but while he lay in a hospital bed in the vascular surgery ward. His dialysis nurse had wheeled him upstairs at the request of his kidney doctor, who had discovered that the arteries in Louie's legs had ceased to function. The same process that had choked off the blood supply to his kidneys now left Louie's feet similarly starved for blood. His toes had turned a dusky shade of blue-black—a color of skin I had never seen.

Surgeons gathered around the end of Louie's bed, pressed and palpated for pulses, and shook their heads when they didn't find any. I stood quietly at the periphery and watched. Once the surgeons decided that Louie would need to stay in the hospital for several days, his dialysis nurse nudged me. Before she left her patient to return to the outpatient dialysis unit, she wanted to outline the intricacies of taking care of Louie. From memory, she recalled the instructions listed on the sheet of paper taped on the counter in the dialysis center.

"Good luck," she said as she left Louie's hospital room. I couldn't tell whether she directed her comment at Louie or at me.

It didn't matter that Louie had ventured out of familiar territory—he still reigned over his kingdom with a strong hand.

"Boy, bring me that paper," he said.

I admonished myself, knowing that the nurse had mentioned Louie's fondness for the newspaper. I wanted to make him smile, and I selfishly hoped for a small acknowledgment that my actions had somehow brightened Louie's day.

"Pull that sheet down a little farther so my toes are covered. No, farther!" And I would jump to pull the sheet down, or draw the shade, or lower the volume of the television.

Under normal circumstances, the hospital staff—me included—would have written off Louie as a "needy" patient. In this case, the tables had turned: Louie capitalized on my eagerness to please and on my lowly rank, and he used it to demonstrate his authority. In this way, despite his short tether to the medical system, he still exerted—and displayed to all—his independence.

Later that evening during rounds, the surgery team discussed the fate of Louie's legs. A number of tests confirmed everyone's worst fear: if we did not amputate *both* of his legs the next morning, Louie ran the risk of developing a fatal infection. The surgeons had already presented Louie with his grim options, and he had willingly consented to the surgery.

After rounds concluded, the surgical team sent me back to perform a preoperative physical examination and told me that unless solicited, I should not speak so much as a word about Louie's impending operation. The surgical resident explained that Louie had specifically asked that no one talk about the events planned for the following day. As I walked toward his room to check his vital signs, the soft sounds of someone crying caused me to stop abruptly at his doorway. I deliberately waited in the hallway until the sniffling had stopped, and then I went in and finished my exam.

Louie laid on the gurney and stared at the ceiling as we rolled him down the hall the following morning. No one spoke a word. Once past the swinging double doors of the operating room, several of us tried to help Louie climb onto the operating table. He furiously slapped our hands away.

"I can do it myself! Just let me take my time, okay?"

Leg by leg, the proud man painstakingly hoisted himself onto the operating table. We tried to stand by nonchalantly, but the concerned looks on our faces would not have fooled anyone. Louie was not in any real danger of falling as he lifted himself onto the table. I think my fear stemmed more from imagining what would happen to Louie's legs after he made it up there.

As soon as Louie was anesthetized, we began to perform what would become the most memorable operation I would witness during my surgery rotation. As each limb fell into the specimen bag that waited below the operating table, I watched Louie's fiercely defended independence mingle with the wisps of putrid Bovie smoke and then vanish.

Two hours later, we lifted Louie back onto the gurney, although this time he did not object. While the surgeons rolled him out of the operating room, I stayed behind to tie up the specimen bags and prepare them for the pathologist. As I picked them up, the heft of the bags caught me completely off guard—I wondered where his legs had traveled and how Louie would possibly tolerate life without them.

That afternoon, I avoided performing Louie's postoperative examination until the last possible moment. Still carrying the weight of his legs in my mind, I did not want to see the look on his face during his darkest moment. To both of our advantages, Louie still had plenty of narcotics in his system, so he dozed while I performed a cursory examination of his heart, lungs, and two, new wounds. As I peeked under the sheet covering Louie's stumps, I felt my face contort. After I left the hospital that night, I stood in front of my bathroom mirror and practiced the next day's greeting.

"How are you doing today?"

No, too normal.

"How was your breakfast?"

No, too upbeat.

"Good morning, sir."

That sounded appropriate enough. I made sure I'd said it fifty times without wincing or contorting before I went to bed.

Despite the preparation, my nerves got the better of me the following morning once I approached Louie's room. I froze in my tracks the moment he looked up from behind his big, thick eyeglasses and locked his eyes with mine. He took the lead.

"Morning, boy," he said. In that instant, I knew by the soft tone of his voice that he would be okay.

"Hey, pull that sheet down over my legs. It's kind of cold in here," he continued. So I pulled the sheet farther down the bed, and neither of us flinched at the absent tents of fabric that his toes would have created. For the first time since we'd met, my actions felt natural and un-orchestrated, and I was motivated by nothing more than a fundamental desire to ease Louie's suffering. Almost instinctively, I adjusted his tray table so that he could reach his bowl of steaming broth, and I set his morning paper in front of him. As the sun came up and began to illuminate the room in a brilliant red, I think that—just for a moment—Louie let down his guard and smiled lovingly on his kingdom.

CHAPTER THIRTY

HEART

"**A**RE YOU READY?" asked Dr. Goldstein.
The woman nodded as the orderly lifted the ornate pillow off its resting place on her chest. The patient's church group had assembled the pillow by hand, in the shape of a heart, to convey their sentiments of support and love. I knew the shape also had literal meaning—the woman was scheduled to have open-heart surgery this morning. Ellen Shaw, this young mother of three, had recurrent pheochromocytoma—a malignant cancer that I had only read about in textbooks. In this condition, the tumor secretes adrenaline that causes panic attacks, raises blood pressure, and places a tremendous burden on a patient's heart. Sometimes the tumor spreads, and it infiltrates and destroys everything in its path. Ellen's tumor had encased her heart (an unusual presentation of this disease) and caused it to beat irregularly. Her surgeons had operated on her three times without improvement, and she didn't flinch while the orderly prepared to wheel her to her fourth, and last, open-heart surgery. Dr. Goldstein, her cardiothoracic surgeon, was clear that if this surgery did not slow her disease, she would be an unlikely candidate for future operations.

As evidenced by the collage of pictures that covered the walls of her hospital room, Ellen's three children provided her with all the strength she needed. I felt a pang of grief as I thought back to Gina. By now, I imagined that she had probably died and left her two children behind. Motherless. What an awful word.

"I'm ready," Ellen said, having gathered the courage to part with her heart-shaped pillow. "Let's go before I change my mind."

The orderly wheeled her down the hallway toward the operating suite, and the rest of us scuttled onward to finish rounds so that everyone could prepare for Ellen's marathon-length surgery. One door down, we visited with John, who suffered from mesothelioma, the same cancer that had killed Ellie. He couldn't have been more than fifty-five years old. John's cancer—although of a different type than Ellen's tumor—had also disseminated throughout his chest and crept into every crevice of his lung.

Carefully, with the door just barely cracked open, we filed into his room one by one. Inside, John sat alone in his dark room with his sunglasses on (the big, wraparound kind that my grandparents wore), afraid to expose himself to any light. His particular type of chemotherapy worked like a Trojan horse: the chemical circulated throughout his body, but was activated only under certain conditions (in his case, by a certain wavelength of light). In the operating room, the cardiothoracic surgeons could slice open his chest and shine the light directly on to the cancer containing parts of his lungs to kill the tumor. At the same time, it made the remainder of his body especially sensitive to visible light. If he did not keep himself secluded until the chemotherapy filtered out of his system, the chemotherapy could cause the cancer to develop elsewhere in his body. Thus, he remained in his tiny room cut off from the rest of the world by his blinds, the drape over his door, and his sunglasses. Each time we squeezed into John's room, I wondered how he tolerated living under these restrictions.

That morning, we stood around his bed orienting ourselves and listening to his ever-hopeful voice cut through the dreary darkness. We could hear him fumbling as he looked for something.

"Here. I got a new picture of my granddaughter," John said.

We could barely see a thing. But after a few moments, my eyes adjusted and I saw the faint outline of a child's beaming smile. The situation seemed utterly unfair: John barely had enough light to make out the beloved subjects in his snapshots—the same people who had provided him with the impetus and strength to undergo the darkness-requiring treatments in the first place. Yet, as we passed the picture around, I felt that—even in the darkness—each of the tough surgeons smiled for a moment and recognized the incredible strength of the man lying before us. Although I couldn't see him, I knew that John was smiling, too, from behind his cloak of darkness.

After we left John's room, the entire team gathered in the operating suite. A crowd had assembled outside the room where Ellen's surgery would take place. The surgeons entered the operating room, while the rest of us observed the surgery on two gigantic LCD screens. For the next fourteen hours, Dr. Goldstein and his team of surgeons performed a tag-team operation, relieving one another for a break after each hour of intense surgery. Every time one of the surgeons walked out of the operating room for a pit stop at the bathroom, a glass of orange juice, or simply to rub the tension from his temples, he appeared distracted and eager to return to his patient.

I saw the surgeons slice open the pericardium, the sack surrounding the actual heart muscle. I saw Ellen's heart stop beating as they pumped her blood out of her body and through the bypass machine. I watched anxiously as the surgeons separated, then nearly lifted, Ellen's heart from her chest and as they scraped the visible tumor from around her heart. I saw the resignation in the surgeons' faces as they begrudgingly placed the organ back into its resting place—with sizeable pockets of unreachable tumor still encasing her heart.

The next day we visited Ellen during morning rounds. I found it difficult to believe that just the day before the surgeons had stopped Ellen's heart from beating while they performed her operation. Today she looked completely fine—smiling, vital, and wondering when she'd go home.

"Ellen, we couldn't get all of it," Dr. Goldstein said after a few moments of silence.

"I didn't expect you to," she replied, smiling.

"I did," he said.

"Maybe you should have been a priest," she said. Then, considering his last name, she jokingly added, "Or a rabbi. You seem to believe in miracles."

As we conducted our postoperative exam, Ellen appeared satisfied with the outcome of her latest surgery. She seemed more pleased than her surgeons did. After we finished, she hugged her heart-shaped pillow close to her chest, which hid her zipper line of suture marks, and then she smiled broadly as her family filed back into the room.

From the look of muted joy in Ellen's eyes, I knew that she knew she'd be back to the hospital again, probably sometime soon. But I also sensed that somehow it didn't matter. Ellen had endured treatments that she knew were only temporary fixes, yet somehow she still managed to maintain a fierce determination to fight her cancer for as long as she could. Like her next-door neighbor John, Ellen would do anything to spend precious moments with her family.

EMERGENCY MEDICINE

CHAPTER THIRTY-ONE

ALL OR NOTHING

MY OWN EXIT from the surgical world was also marked with smiles, albeit for a less somber reason than Ellen's was. Although I was thankful to have seen that side of medicine, I knew the practice of surgery was not for me. From what I had observed, it demanded too much effort to maintain a life both inside and outside the world of the hospital. And with the end of third year only two weeks away, I did not intend to make any career decisions—finishing the year was momentous enough.

For my final rotation, I was excited to return to a familiar place: the ER. Throughout the year, I had noticed that the ER was the one common denominator for each of the rotations. Doctors from every medical discipline—internal medicine or obstetrics or surgery—admitted patients through the ER. By the time I started my ER clerkship, I had already experienced my fair share of emergency medicine and I felt excited—not anxious—to begin the rotation. Whether it was true evidence that I had settled into the role of a medical student or a false sense of security because of my familiarity with the ER, I still felt confident as I concluded the third year of medical school with two weeks of emergency medicine.

Two residents called out sick my first night in the ER. The nurses and the attending physicians seemed to think this equaled a catastrophic event—for me, it meant an opportunity to gain plenty of hands-on experience. Within the first twenty minutes, I performed my first chest compression.

Using an old, handheld walkie-talkie, the ER attending physician communicated with a paramedic about an inbound patient.

"Seventy-year-old man. Likely myocardial infarction," crackled the voice over the radio. "Intubated in the field. Estimated time of arrival is less than five minutes."

When the paramedics burst through the door with the patient, we learned that someone had found him slumped on a park bench. By the time the paramedics had arrived, the man did not have a palpable pulse, and the paramedics had started chest compressions. Before arriving at the hospital, they had also inserted a plastic breathing tube into his trachea—no small feat outside the controlled environment of the hospital. As soon as we had lifted the patient off the transport gurney and onto the ER stretcher, the attending physician started barking orders.

"Get a line in," he yelled. "Pull up some epinephrine. Let's go."

The paramedic continued to perform compressions.

"Get ready, med student," said the attending physician. I was next in line to relieve the paramedic when his arms tired. While I waited, I tried to remember the number of compressions I was supposed to perform for each breath delivered by the person in charge of the patient's airway. Fifteen-to-one? Thirty-to-two?

"In five, med student," the attending physician said before I could come up with the right answer. Sadly, I had learned to respond to the phrase "med student" as if it was my given name, but right then was not the time to lament that fact.

I took a deep breath, stepped up on the stool beside the table for leverage to perform adequate compressions, and traded places with the paramedic. Pressing with the full force of my upper body, I started counting. What surprised me the most was the amount of force needed to compress a human chest. I met significant resistance as I pushed with my palms.

"Harder, deeper, longer," I heard the attending physician yelling from behind me. Had I not been learning how to perform CPR on a real patient, I may have keeled over in laughter—the attending physician sounded like a director of an adult movie. I followed his instructions, pushing harder against the man's chest. I felt crunching from beneath my hands, followed by a decrease in the resistance after I had broken several ribs. In my CPR manual, I had read that broken ribs were a normal—and sometimes necessary—part of CPR, but I never expected to break someone's ribs. Nonetheless, I continued to administer compressions until my shoulder and back muscles burned with fatigue. Another medical student, one of my friends also working in the ER, relieved me. I stepped back from the scene, my head filled with awful images, and promptly felt sick to my stomach. I left the resuscitation bay, worried that I might vomit, and I sat down to calm the waves of nausea.

About ten minutes later, a stream of people filtered out of the man's room. The man was dead. Technically, the man had not been alive for some time—probably not since suffering a heart attack on the park bench. I thought the attending physician probably realized this since he had two medical students perform a key portion of the resuscitation, which was more responsibility than I had been granted during the past year. As the attending physician debriefed us about the event, he confirmed this point: "Don't beat yourselves up about it. This man was not going to survive, regardless of the care he received. He was dead when he came through the door." I hoped to God that he was right; I was sure that I had inflicted the pain of several broken ribs on the man.

I had a difficult time falling asleep that night. I kept imagining the sound of his crunching ribs. For the next two days, I walked around on the constant verge of vomiting, and I avoided anything that hinted at the idea of death. On my subsequent nights in the ER, I felt thankful that none of the residents called out sick. It meant that I fell from being a starting player to a pinch hitter, but that was fine with me for a few days.

———

Several shifts into my rotation, I had an incredible experience that reminded me how small the world could be. The paramedics arrived with another man whom they had found slumped on a park bench, but I entered the resuscitation bay to find that this man had a pulse—he would fare better than my last patient.

I started to help the nurses cut off the man's layers of clothing (which, I had started to learn, signaled that he lived on the street). Beneath the patient's salt-and-pepper stubble, I recognized the unmistakable face of Andre Benson, one of the first—and feistiest—patients I had cared for at the beginning of my third year of medical school.

Almost an entire year had passed since I stood beside his bed that terrifying, first day of my internal medicine rotation and listened to the resident spout-off foreign acronyms: PT, PTT, PE, DVT. I remembered that Mr. Benson's right leg had developed a massive blood clot, a piece of which had broken off and lodged itself in one of the major arteries in his lung. He had grown ornery and inpatient as we tried—unsuccessfully—to thin his blood with medicine. Although I had rotated on to another clerkship by the time his medical team discharged him from the hospital, I had assumed Mr. Benson would be fine. After his close brush with death, I believed he would adhere to the team's recommendations.

Looking at him lying on the gurney cocooned within layers of threadbare rags, sad disappointment overcame me. I knew it made no sense to personalize this patient, but somehow I felt as though Mr. Benson had failed me. The smell of his breath suggested that he had not kicked his alcohol problem. I didn't want to consider the necessary medications he probably wasn't taking, including his blood-thinning Coumadin.

The attending physician must have noticed the surprised expression on my face, and I explained how I knew the homeless man.

"Ah, so you must know how headstrong Mr. Benson can be," he replied, unsurprised by my comment. Clearly, he had taken care of Mr. Benson before, which reinforced how insignificant the care I had provided back on the medicine ward must have seemed in this man's life. He was a frequent flyer in the ER, and only my naïveté made me think the concern and campaigning I had done on his behalf would change his life.

"He's almost always drunk. Rarely, if ever, does he want any of our help. In fact, all he ever needs is a refill on his pills," the attending physician continued. He formed quotation marks with his fingers to emphasize the absurdity of this last statement. Hearing these stories about Mr. Benson's stubborn behavior helped alleviate my frustration.

Our ER team decided Mr. Benson would be just fine with some basic care, such as rehydrating him, allowing him to sober up, and just to be safe, running a few basic blood tests. When the laboratory test results came back about an hour later, one of the numbers caught my eye. His INR, a measure of the blood's tendency to clot, was well within the range signifying adequate anticoagulation. Mr. Benson *had* followed the one instruction that the medical team had emphasized above all else—he had properly taken his blood thinning medication. An overwhelming sense of awe replaced my feelings of frustration, anger, and disappointment.

I had been so focused on my own unfair expectations of Mr. Benson that I neglected to consider the humble progress he had made within the context of his life. In doing so, I took my perceptions of Mr. Benson's "failures" too personally, and I approached him with an unwarranted resentment. His medication history notwithstanding, I should have first celebrated his success in keeping the one promise he'd made to himself—to spend a little more time in this world—and that he'd done it despite the harsh, unrelenting conditions of life on the street.

The experience caused me to reflect on some unsettled and unresolved feelings I first encountered while caring for Alden, the patient who had walked out of the hospital against medical advice. For most of the past year, I continued to question myself whether, as a medical professional, I could legitimately feel anger toward my patients. Every time the issue surfaced, I pushed the emotion back down and ignored it. Today was the first time I found evidence—real, undeniable proof—of the danger in expecting too much from a patient and then faulting him when he didn't live up to his potential.

As I reminisced about all the patients I had cared for during the last year, I realized that in more than a few instances, I had unfairly judged many of them—such as Alden, or the young couple who gave up their son for adoption, or Edward, the schizophrenic patient—without first considering all of the information. If I hadn't initially set such high expectations, I might have provided more compassionate care to them.

My encounter with Mr. Benson reinforced that I couldn't expect patients to move forward at my pace—I needed to move at theirs. Sometimes people made progress in leaps and bounds, like Edward had, and sometimes they moved at a snail's pace, as in the case of Alden. Subsequently, I realized the importance of evaluating progress not as an all-or-nothing phenomenon, but as a series of gradual steps along a continuum between those two extremes. Mr. Benson humbly reminded me, with just a slight shift in thinking, how momentous each of those steps could be, once I recognized the net effect as movement forward.

CHAPTER THIRTY-TWO

A FEW GRAY HAIRS

THE ELDERLY WOMAN'S EYELIDS grew heavy, and then mid-sentence, her head drooped to one side and loud snoring filled the room. I decided our interaction must have bored her enough that she had fallen asleep. I laughed to myself and wondered if she did the same to her daughter who had brought her to the ER. I imagined the small, frail woman feigning sleep every time she wanted to tune out the world.

Her daughter had grown worried because her mother seemed more confused lately. At first, her daughter thought the confusion marked the inevitable beginning of Alzheimer's disease. But earlier that day, her mother had taken a sudden turn for the worse, and she slipped in and out of consciousness. I took the daughter's concern seriously. Altered mental status—the medical term for inappropriate confusion or sleepiness—had a large number of important possible causes, some of which, such as stroke, had grave prognoses.

Once the attending physician in the ER had cleared the elderly woman from having any immediately life-threatening conditions, he sent me back into the room do a more thorough history and physical. I wanted to see if I could come up with a diagnosis and plan by myself. I began to have a brief conversation with the elderly woman, but she decided to tune me out again, and I finished the interview by speaking with her daughter.

"Has she been taking any new medications?"

"No."

"Has she complained of any fluttering in her chest?"

"No."

For the next ten minutes, I went through a long list of causes of altered mental status, and I asked all the relevant questions. My verbal investigation turned up nothing. Imagining myself as a private eye of sorts, I decided to see if I could find any other physical clues. Starting with the elderly woman's frail body, I searched for telltale signs: an irregular heartbeat, a twitching muscle, or a wandering eye. Again, my search yielded nothing. Resorting to the equivalent of sifting through someone's garbage can, I commandeered the elderly woman's handbag from her daughter and rifled through its contents. Half a dozen brown prescription containers spilled from the purse. I checked each one to make sure that her daughter faithfully recalled each medication's name and dosing schedule, which she had. Then, near the bottom of the purse, I noticed a small cardboard box, the same kind of container that houses over-the-counter medications in the pharmacy—it was labeled "URISTAT." Interesting.

"Has your mother complained of any pain with urination over the last few days?" I asked the daughter.

"Now that I think about it, she did say she had a bit of burning, but nothing too out of the ordinary," she replied. "URISTAT normally seems to take care of it."

Echoing in the back of my mind was the mantra I'd heard a million times during the last year, "Common things are common." Then, a little lightbulb flashed in my head—urinary tract infections were the most common cause of altered mental status in the elderly population. In my mind, the diagnosis was as good as gold, so I asked the daughter if she could help her mother fill a specimen cup with urine.

Five minutes later, standing in the small ER laboratory, I hunched over the counter and waited for the urine test strip to develop. The strip had several small marks along its length that changed color depending on the presence or absence of certain chemicals in a patient's urine. Then, using a decoder, I interpreted the strip's color combination to determine if the patient had a urinary tract infection. Purple, green, red, red, purple—positive!

Having made my first bona fide, solo diagnosis, I experienced a new sense of pride—I had worked up the case from the beginning and clinched the diagnosis myself. Although it was not the kind of diagnosis to write home about, it nevertheless made me think that I could handle this doctor thing after all. I tracked down the attending physician to dazzle him with my diagnostic abilities.

"Cut to the chase," he instructed me, gruffly. "Just give me your assessment and problem list."

"Well, she is an eighty-year-old woman who lives at home with her daughter. She has a one-day history of altered mental status. She has a positive urine dip. I believe her symptoms are secondary to a urinary tract infection," I said. "I'd like to give her a dose of antibiotic here, make sure her condition improves, and then discharge her home."

"Anything else?"

"She should follow up with her primary care doctor in a day or two?" I said, unsure about what other details I could provide. It seemed by the book to me.

"What are you forgetting?"

"Umm," I said, trying to buy time. "I don't know."

"Go get me a phone book," he instructed.

A phone book?

Reluctantly, I trudged across the ER to the receptionist's desk and asked for a phone book. She forked over the thick volume, which I grudgingly lugged back across the ER and attempted to hand to the attending physician.

"No, this is for you," the attending physician said. "You're the one who's going to need it. What's on the back cover?"

Baffled, I flipped it over.

"Right there in front of your eyes. What's that say across the back cover?"

"Lehman and Lehman, LLC. We fight for you," I recited, reading the caption from an advertisement for a local ambulance-chasing law firm.

"You're not going to survive in this business for very long unless you practice 'CYA medicine,'" he lectured. I'd never heard the term "CYA medicine" before.

"Cover your ass," he said. "You need to cover your ass, or you'll never make it through residency. What if your old lady has altered mental status because of a prescription drug overdose? Or because she was having an acute aortic dissection? Or because she was high on crack? They'd take away those two letters after your name before you'd have the chance to use them."

I'd performed a thorough physical exam, and both the attending physician and the CT scan had ruled out a stroke as a possibility. I'd thought about the life-threatening possibilities. But in this particular situation, the evidence hadn't supported any of them as real contenders. I wanted to yell at him, "It's a simple urinary tract infection!" Instead, I laughed to myself at the absolute absurdity of his statement, and I imagined the tiny, eighty-year-old woman plodding behind her walker toward the local street corner so she could refill her marijuana supply.

After the attending physician finished lecturing me about the dangers of not practicing CYA medicine, I followed him back into my patient's room, and he performed his own history and physical.

"The urine dip was positive?" he asked me, while he examined her reflexes.

"Yes."

"I'd like to treat her with an antibiotic for a urinary tract infection," he explained to the patient's daughter. "We'll give her a dose here, and then you can fill the rest of the prescription at your pharmacy. If anything comes up in the meantime—fever, chest pain, or slurred speech—then you should bring your mother back to the ER."

The daughter thanked the attending physician, but I ignored him and walked out of the room to let off some steam. If the last several months of surgery had taught me anything, it was to let go of things out of my control. Today, I felt proud that I had made my first diagnosis, even if it was the simplest of diagnoses. After I located an empty bathroom (which, over the past year, I had discovered was the one place where I could *always* find solitude), I stood in front of the mirror and noticed I had acquired a few gray hairs on either side of my head. I looked at myself, and I wondered whether the gray hairs served only as a measure of the stress I experienced during the past year, or if they also reflected my growth into a more seasoned—and slightly wiser—medical student.

During the last week of my third year of medical school, one of the deans contacted me to see if I would show some of the soon to be third year medical students around the hospital. I agreed and decided that I would take them to see a few patients, walk them through writing a patient progress note, and answer any questions they might have before starting their upcoming rotations.

Later that night, after returning home from another shift in the ER, I sent an e-mail to the three students whom the dean had assigned to me. I provided them with directions to the ER, my pager number, and remembering my own initial experience in the hospital, explicit instructions on how to use the paging system. The e-mail read, "Dial the pager number, wait for the beeps, punch in your phone number, and then hit '#.' Make sure to hang around long enough to answer the phone, so that you can talk with the person you paged."

A few days later, after our agreed-on meeting time had come and then passed, I repeatedly checked my beeper and wondered why the students hadn't paged me yet. Figuring the students were probably just running late from class, I went to see another patient. After I emerged from the exam room, I noticed several confused-looking people lingering around the nurses' station. Their short white coats gave them away immediately.

Before rescuing them, I studied the scene. I envisioned what my supervising resident must have seen that first day—almost a full year ago—when she found me at the nurses' station. One of the medical students, while holding a phone to her ear, clenched her free hand into a fist and then swiped it through the air in a "damn-it" motion. The two other students stood staring at a crumpled piece of paper trying to figure out where they had gone wrong.

"Hi, guys," I said, smiling. I inquired whether they were the medical students the dean had assigned to me. They looked at me with frightened, pleading eyes and nodded.

"Don't worry. The first time I ever tried to page someone, I failed miserably, too. Almost made me decide to quit medical school right there and then," I said. Then, I took a few minutes to demonstrate how the paging system worked and noticed the worry in their eyes slowly recede.

During the course of the next several hours, I introduced the students to the sights, smells, and sounds of the hospital wards. I pointed out where the patient charts were stored and helped them write a sample admission note. I showed them the places they could sneak away to when they needed a quiet minute, recited the cafeteria hours, and told them just about everything I thought might make their transition a bit easier. They took it all in, wide-eyed and nodding, still mostly at a loss for words. Then, as we finished the tour, the quietest of the three students spoke up.

"How did you learn so much so quickly? I mean, you're only a year ahead of us, but you're practically a *real* doctor!"

The statement caught me a bit off-guard. To be honest, until that moment, I hadn't seen myself as anything other than a slightly less-bumbling-and-incompetent version of the medical student who stood in their shoes just a year before. I paused, trying to think of how to respond to the question. Then it came to me. And it seemed so simple.

"It just kind of—" I hesitated, thinking my answer was too clichéd. But I decided that it *was* the truth. "Well, it really just kind of happened."

They smiled and seemed surprisingly satisfied with my response.

I smiled, too. Without knowing it, they had just given me the answers to questions that I had asked myself repeatedly over the past year: Would I ever have what it takes to become a doctor? Would I ever fit into that long white coat?

Yes, I decided.

Yes, I would.

GLOSSARY

ACL. Anterior cruciate ligament, a fibrous band within the knee.

Admission. When a patient is admitted to a room in the hospital; also known as the bane of a resident's existence.

Attending physician. The most senior doctor on the team, the commander in chief.

Bovie. A surgical instrument that burns through tissue; also responsible for creating the medical student's job of holding a suction catheter for hours on end in the operating room to remove the smell.

Bronchoscopy. A procedure in which a fiber-optic tube is guided into a patient's airway to examine for lung disease.

Call night. The painful hours of 5:00 PM to 7:00 AM, when a resident is responsible for all of a medical team's patients, as well as any new admissions to the hospital.

CBC. Complete blood count, a test to measure types of cells in a patient's body.

CHF. Congestive heart failure, a form of heart failure in which the heart cannot pump effectively and fluid builds up in the body, including in the lungs.

Code. When someone is actively trying to die.

CPS. Child Protective Services, the agency responsible for investigating all cases of child abuse and neglect.

Creatinine. A blood test to measure the kidneys' ability to function.

CT scan. Computed tomography, a method of obtaining three-dimensional imaging of the body.

DNR. Do not resuscitate, meaning that a patient has opted to forgo any specified life-saving measures.

DVT. Deep venous thrombosis, a blood clot in a large vein, usually in a leg.

EKG. Electrocardiogram, a way to examine the structure and function of the heart.

ER. Emergency room.

Foley. A type of catheter that is inserted in the urethra to help a patient urinate; a painful procedure for both patients and doctors.

HIV. Human immunodeficiency virus, the virus that leads to AIDS.

ICU. Intensive care unit, where patients can be monitored closely because of a higher ratio of nurses to patients.

INR. International normalized ratio, a standardized way of measuring the blood's ability to clot that is frequently used to monitor the success of anticoagulation.

Intern. A first-year resident who has finished medical school and received his medical license; similar to a deer caught in headlights.

IV. Intravenous line, a conduit to deliver fluid and medications directly into a patient's venous system.

Medical student. A person in medical school who has not yet received his medical license; everyone's bitch.

OB-GYN. Obstetrics and gynecology, a male medical student's worst nightmare.

Pimping. The demeaning process of asking a medical student to answer a series of impossible-to-answer questions.

PT and PTT. Prothrombin time and partial prothrombin time, both are measures of the blood's ability to clot.

Pulmonary embolism. A blood clot that blocks major arteries in the lungs and effectively cuts off the blood supply; often occurs in patients with DVT's.

Resident. A physician who has completed intern year and decided to continue the punishment for another year.

Running the numbers. A medical-style piano recital of various patient parameters such as vital signs, laboratory values, and urine/vomit/stool output.

Scut work. Anything that needs to be done, usually menial tasks such as fetching coffee for the team or recording the volume of a patient's stool output.

Speculum. The reason male medical students hate OB-GYN; also why female patients hate male medical students.

Stat. Get your ass in gear—this one's important.

Stool. The nice word for poop.

Troponin. A chemical marker of a recent heart attack.

Ward. A place in the hospital where patient rooms are located.

About the Author

James A. Feinstein, MD, survived medical school and now thrives as a practicing pediatrician. After graduating from Dartmouth College with a degree in biochemistry and molecular biology, he obtained his medical degree from the University of Pennsylvania School of Medicine. He completed an internship in pediatrics at Seattle Children's Hospital before returning to the Children's Hospital of Philadelphia to finish his residency training. His prose has won numerous writing awards, and his short stories have been published in multiple journals. When he is not doctoring or writing, he spends his time in the outdoors, climbing mountains with his best friend and wife, Amy.

CPSIA information can be obtained
at www.ICGtesting.com
Printed in the USA
LVHW091944280619
622692LV00001B/1/P
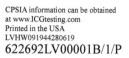

9 781440 175152